MOTHER NATURE'S
MEDICINE CABINET

A to Z Reference Guide For Beginners.

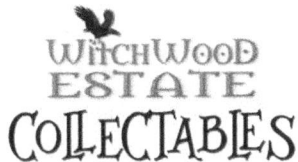

Witchwood Estate Collectables.

Book 3

> *"Let thy food be thy medicine and thy medicine be thy food."* -
> *Hippocrates (460-377 B.C.)*

PATTI ROBERTS

Visit Patti's Facebook page: http://on.fb.me/1waO1jO

Make sure you join my newsletter and be kept up to date on new releases, special promotions, and freebies.

JOIN UP FOR PATTI ROBERTS NEWSLETTER:
http://bit.ly/PattiRobertsNewsletter

First Printing: January 2018
© Cover design by Paradox Designs Covers & Formatting.
https://goo.gl/JNyHHC

Publications by Patti Roberts

eBooks - Freebies.
Once Were Friends.
A 20k prologue to Whoever Said Love Was Easy?

Witchwood Estate Collectables
The Witches' Journal – book 1.
Diffusing Essential Oils - book 2

Writing Tips From Authors.
Believe.
Witchwood Estate – Going Home – (book 1) FREE
Paradox – The Angels Are Here (book 1) FREE

Witchwood Estate
Witchwood Estate – Going Home – (book 1) FREE
Witchwood Estate – Ferntree Falls
Witchwood Estate – Print Edition (book 1 and 2)
Witchwood Estate – Cursed (book 3)
Witchwood Estate – Timeless (book 4)
Witchwood Estate – Witches Bitches (book 5)

Paradox Series
Paradox – The Angels Are Here (book 1) 2010 FREE
Paradox – Progeny Of Innocence (book 2)
Paradox – Bound By Blood (book 3)
Paradox – Equilibrium (book 4)
Paradox – Elemental (book 5)
Standalone Novel
Whoever Said Love Was Easy? About Three Authors series

Non-fiction novels
Surviving Tracy – true stories from the survivors of Cyclone Tracy.
My Hero's Journey – Writing Journal. Plot your novel from start to finish – Easy to follow examples. Includes character profiles.
Coming soon
Little Book Of Smoothies: For when your mojo needs a boost! (Witchwood Estate Collectables 4)
http://amzn.to/2Dr27c4
Paradox: Breathe - book 6
Witchwood Estate: Heart Bound book 6
KLA2EEN: First Contact book 1

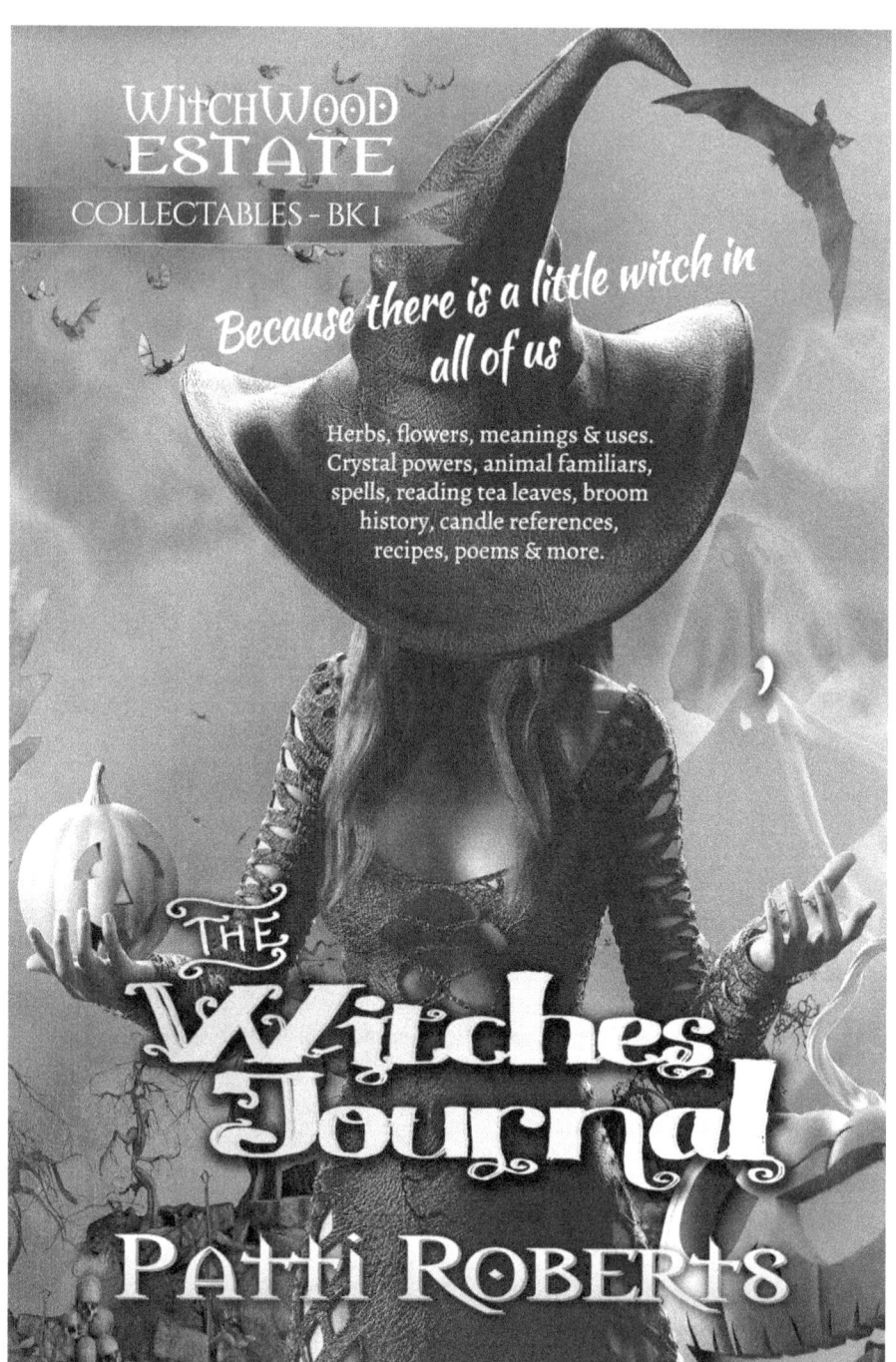

WitchWood
ESTATE
COLLECTABLES - BK 1

Because there is a little witch in all of us

Herbs, flowers, meanings & uses.
Crystal powers, animal familiars,
spells, reading tea leaves, broom
history, candle references,
recipes, poems & more.

THE
Witches
Journal

PATTI ROBERTS

MOTHER NATURE'S MEDICINE CABINET.

Keep all essential oils out of reach from children and pets.

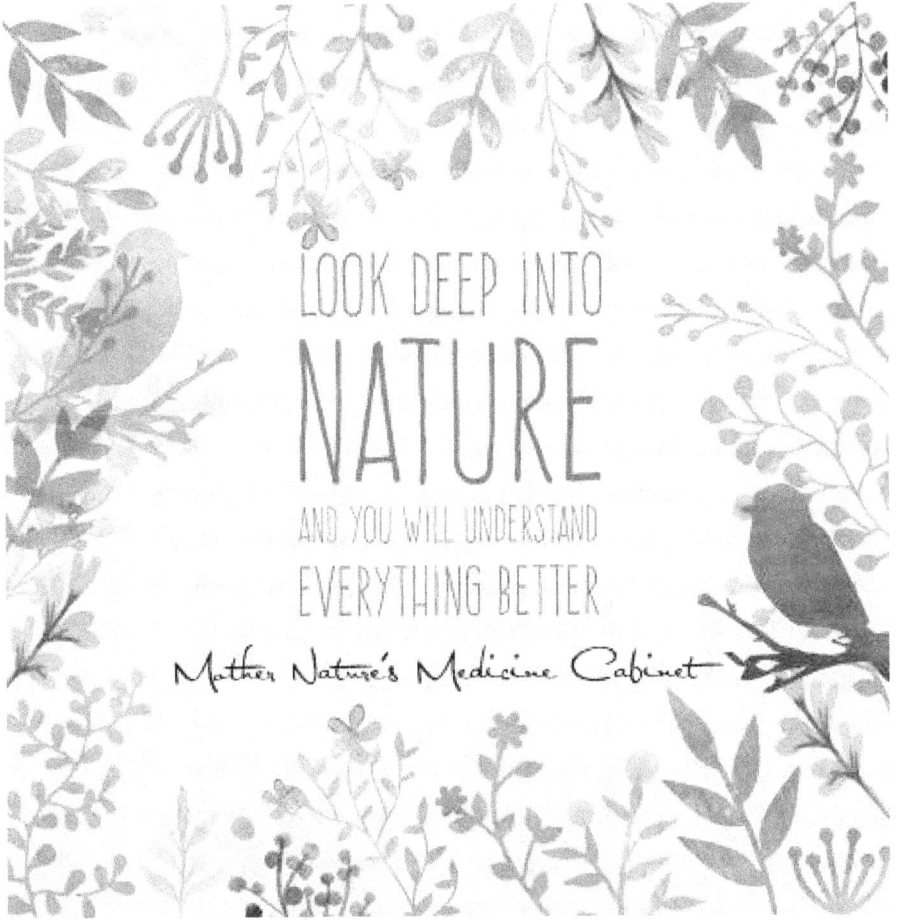

LOOK DEEP INTO NATURE AND YOU WILL UNDERSTAND EVERYTHING BETTER

Mother Nature's Medicine Cabinet

Rid your household of toxic chemicals that are making you sick. There is a healthy alternative. *Mother Nature's Medicine Cabinet* is a handy guide to discovering the natural healing and cleansing powers of essential oils. If you're interested in the topic of essential oils and their many benefits, then this book is for you.

Since ancient times, essential oils have been known to possess natural healing powers—but even natural remedies can cause harm if not used correctly. Knowing how to use essential oils safely around the home is vital to reap the many rewards.

Aromatic plants were the basis for herbal and botanical medicines and remedies for thousands of years - they still are. In fact, they're the root of today's modern pharmaceuticals.

As lifestyles rapidly changed to meet everyday challenges, and technology progressed in leaps and bounds, herbal knowledge soon fell by the wayside. During the past century, as the side effects of many chemically based drugs and cleaning products became known, natural alternatives have found their way back into our homes. People are educating themselves in the uses and the wonderful benefits of using essential oils. Mother nature's medicine cabinet is back, invoking endless remedies - without the toxic side effects.

Natural healing with essential oils may not replace the family doctor or chemically manufactured products entirely, but it most certainly is a healthy alternative to consider when thinking about your family's well-being.

With *Mother Nature's Medicine Cabinet*, you'll quickly discover the heart of what it means to live a healthy and natural lifestyle.

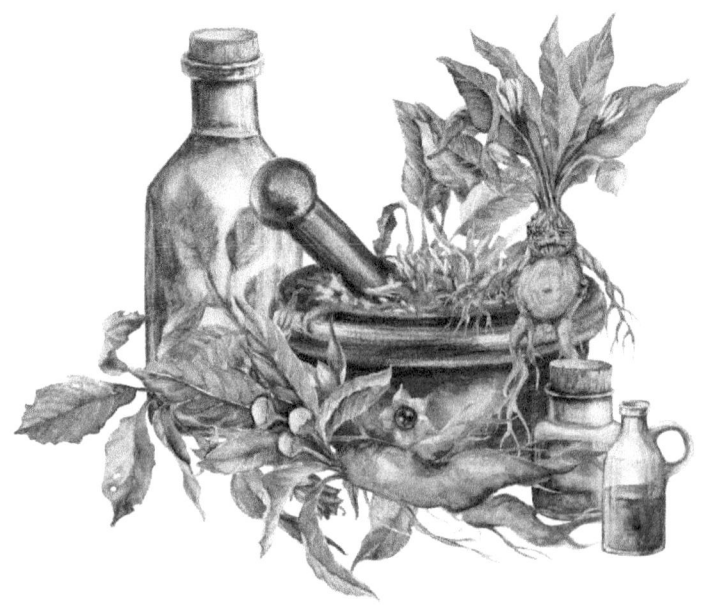

CONTENTS

A NOTE FROM THE AUTHOR.

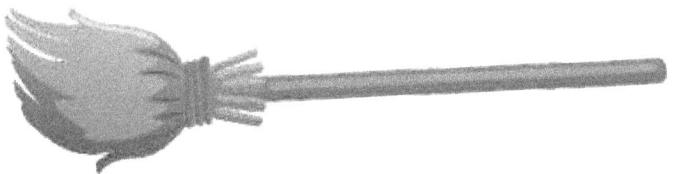

Recently I bought my first diffuser and stocked up on some of my favorite essential oils. I have to say that I'm now hooked on essential oils and their array of uses. I love using my diffuser and use it on a daily basis – night and day. Not only for the lovely aromas but for the health benefits as well.

Not so long ago I used plug-in air fresheners to keep my home smelling nice but having learned of the toxic chemicals used in these products, I have ceased to use them entirely, opting for the healthier and friendlier option.

> *Once I researched all the health benefits associated with using essential oils in diffusers, I decided the next step was to share what I'd learned by compiling the information in the Diffusing Essential Oils.*

Thousands of copies of the free ebook have been downloaded to date. Of course, there are many ways of using essential oils to benefit your health and wellbeing, and this book lists the most popular oils available today. Patti - Check out the facebook page.

DEDICATION

This dedication is to my family and friends, and to all those who purchase and read my books. I trust you will enjoy this one. I would be pleased to hear from you after you read it. pattiroberts7@gmail.com

Dear Readers: All my books go through numerous edits, nonetheless, typos and other errors somehow sometimes survive the process. If you encounter any errors, please send them to me at

pattiroberts7@gmail.com

> *"If we doctors threw all our medicines into the sea, it would be that much better for our patients and that much worse for the fishes."*
> *Supreme Court Justice Oliver Wendel Holmes, MD*

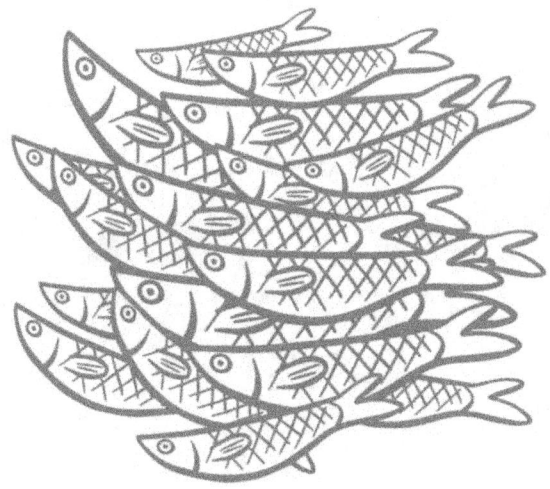

DISCLAIMER.

The information included this book is not intended to diagnose, treat, or prevent any disease. The content I am sharing with you is not intended to be a substitute for professional medical advice. Always seek the advice of a physician or a qualified health professional with any questions you may have regarding specific situations. Any information within this book about the possible health benefits using essential oils have not been evaluated by any Food or Drug Administration.

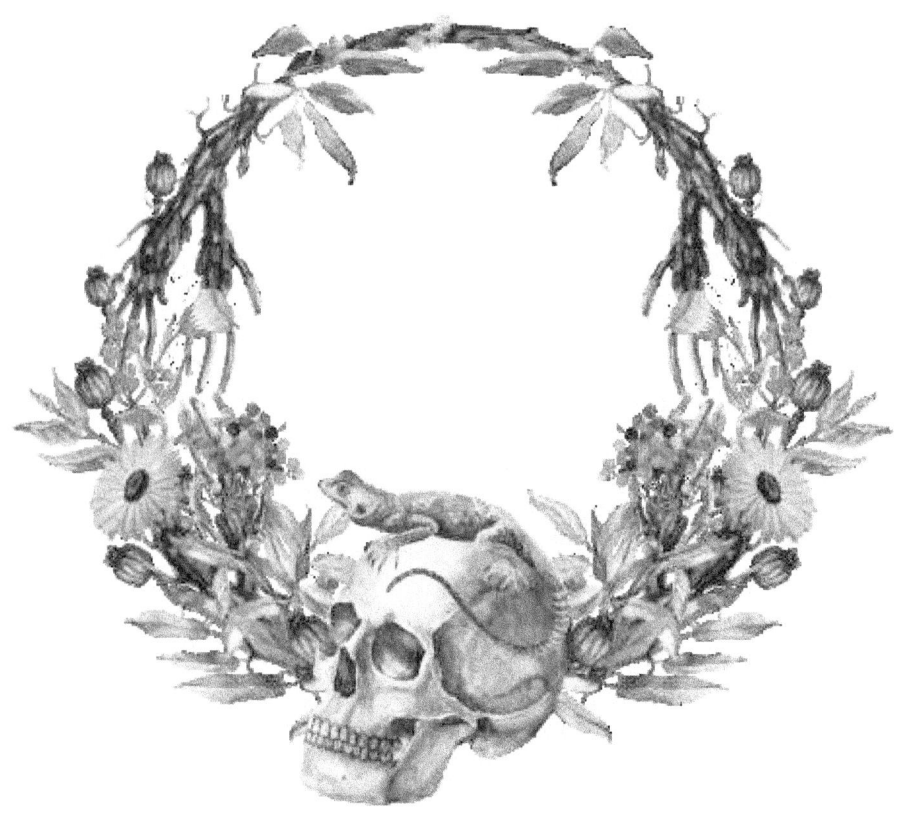

WARNING.

For pet owners, especially those with cats, do not diffuse essential oils in closed, poorly ventilated areas when your pets are in the room. Many essential oils are highly toxic, especially to cats.

Before you start using essential oils, it may be a good idea to do a patch test first to make sure you don't experience any diverse reactions. Especially those who are prone to sensitive skin issues.

It is advised to always keep essential oils out of reach from small children and animals.

Some oils can also be problematic for those with asthma and allergies, so don't go overboard! Essential oils can enter the body in three ways:
- applied directly to the skin.
- inhaled.
- ingested.

With that in mind, there are several kinds of application methods. For example, you can apply essential oils topically in several ways. Such as: Compresses, sprays, diffusers, baths, or massage them into your skin. Make sure you research and only source high-quality (organic if possible) oils from reputable suppliers.

If you are ever in doubt using essential oils, or how to apply them, consult an experienced aromatherapist. Check with your preferred health food store; they usually have an essential oil specialist on hand. Keep in mind that some oils should never be used on babies or young children. Dilution is significantly important when using essential oils. Regardless of the brand you buy, what essential oil you are using, or how much, it is not safe to use any most essential oils neat without first diluting it in a carrier oil or some other type of dilution.

SEVEN BASIC ESSENTIAL OILS TO GET YOU STARTED.

If you haven't already done so, consider adding these six essential oils to your essential medicine cabinet.

Frankincense: Boosts your immune system, reduces inflammation, heals age spots, and supports brain function. Anti-inflammatory, heal bruising, reduce scars, and boosts emotional well-being. Research shows that it may also be helpful in fighting cancer.

Lavender: One of the most commonly used oils, lavender helps with relaxation and sleep. Lowers anxiety, improves mood, and heals burns, cuts, rashes, stings. Lavender restores skin complexion and reduces acne. Slows the aging process with powerful antioxidants. Improves eczema and psoriasis.

Lemon: Perfect to use in homemade cleaning products. It improves lymph drainage and cleanses the body. Nourishes the skin and promotes weight loss. Calms stomach and relieves nausea. Helps to overcome addictions while improving mood to fight depression.

Orange: Antispasmodic. Relaxes muscular and nervous spasms and coughing. Alleviates anxiety, anger, depression, and inflammation. Aphrodisiac properties. Orange aids both fungal infections, septic, and tetanus, and can disinfect the wound. Ideal for people who suffer from depression or chronic anxiety. Helps eliminate houseflies.

Peppermint: Supports in digestion, improves focus, boosts energy, reduces a fever, soothes headaches, and relieves muscle and joint pain. Clear sinuses, improve asthma and bronchitis. Aids weight loss by suppressing cravings. And it smells great in your diffuser.

Rosemary: Respiratory support, memory, digestion, and supports healthy hair and scalp - stimulates hair growth. Disinfectants, anti-inflammatory, carminative, and antibacterial. Lowers anxiety, mental disorders and depression. Pain, headaches and rheumatism. Respiratory problems, including; bronchial asthma, indigestion, and gas. Rosemary also prevents and reduces infection. It cleans the air of pathogens and allergens. Ideal to clear pimples and athletes foot.

Tea tree oil: (Melaleuca): Is a natural anti-bacterial, anti-fungal, and aids in stimulating the immune system. Tea tree oil a valued natural remedy for treating bacterial and fungal skin conditions, preventing infection and promoting healing. Tea tree oil kills or repels bugs. In some cases, it is as effective as commercial insecticides or repellents, making it a healthier alternative. Reduces bad odors.

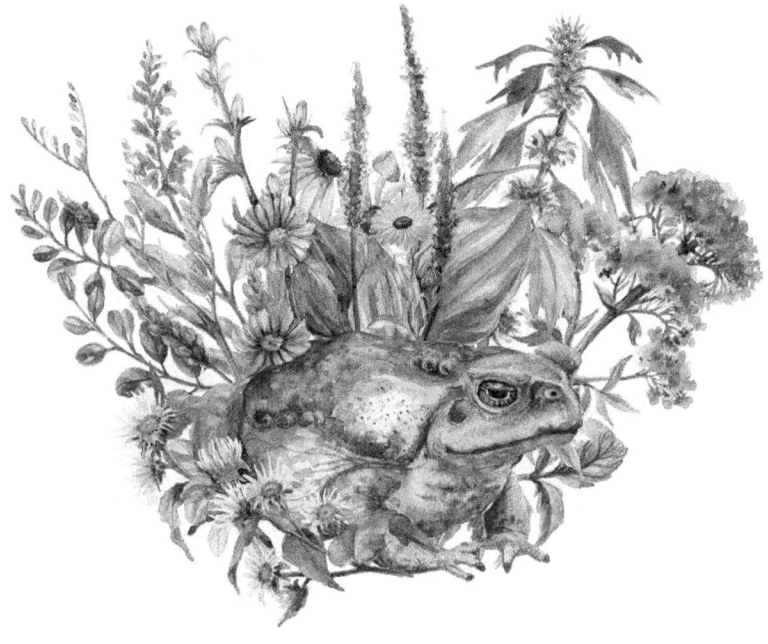

CONVERSION CHARTS

CONVERSION CHART

16 tablespoons	= 1 cup
12 tablespoons	= 3/4 cup
10 tablespoons + 2 teaspoons	= 2/3 cup
8 tablespoons	= 1/2 cup
6 tablespoons	= 3/8 cup
5 tablespoons + 1 teaspoon	= 1/3 cup
4 tablespoons	= 1/4 cup
2 tablespoons	= 1/8 cup
2 tablespoons + 2 teaspoons	= 1/6 cup
1 tablespoon	= 1/16 cup
2 cups	= 1 pint
2 pints	= 1 quart
3 teaspoons	= 1 tablespoon

SPOON CONVERSIONS

Metric to Standard

5 ml................. 1 teaspoon
15 ml............... 1 tablespoon
30 ml............... 1 fluid ounces
240 ml............. 1 cup
1 liter.............. 34 fluid ounces
1 liter.............. 4.2 cups
1 gram............. 0.035 ounce
100 grams........ 3.5 ounces
500 grams........ 1.10 pounds

Cups to Tablespoons

1/8 cup................. 1 tablespoon
1/4 cup................. 2 tablespoons
1/3 cup................. 4 tablespoons
1/2 cup................. 5 tablespoons +
                         1 teaspoon
3/4 cup................. 8 tablespoon
1 cup.................... 16 tablespoon

3 tsp............ 1 Tbsp..... 1/2 ounce.
2 Tbsp......... 1/8 cup.... 1 ounce.
4 Tbsp......... 1/4 cup.... 2 ounces.
5 -1/3 Tbsp... 1/3 cup.... 2.6 ounces.
8 Tbsp......... 1/2 cup.... 4 ounces.
12 Tbsp........ 3/4 cup.... 6 ounces.
16 Tbsp........ 1 cup...... 8 ounces.
32 Tbsp........ 2 cups..... 16 ounces.

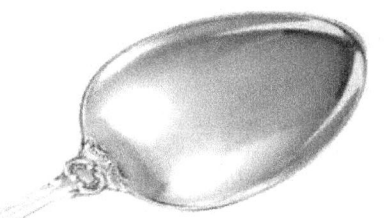

"Until man duplicates a blade of grass, nature can laugh at his so-called scientific knowledge. Remedies from chemicals will never stand in favour compared with the products of nature, the living cell of the plant, the final result of the rays of the sun, the mother of all life." - T. A. Edison

A GUIDE TO DILUTING ESSENTIAL OILS

How much or how little essential oil to use depends on what your intention is. Here is a brief guide to dilution of essential oils.

The active chemical elements found in essential oils can't be denied. They are so powerful in fact that they can cause some very serious health problems if not administered properly. These include: mucolytic irritation, neuro-toxicity, convulsions, skin burning, headaches, discoloration, and dermal sensitivity. Use caution and seek advice when using certain oils on pets, pregnant women, and infants. Failing to do so may lead to illness or even death when swallowed (for particular oils). **It is always important to use caution when handling and applying the oils.**

There are compounds found in essential oils that are toxic when ingested, such as: Boldo, calamus, camphor, horseradish, cassia, pennyroyal, mustard, mugwort, rue, savin, tansy, sassafras, thuja, wintergreen, wormseed, and wormwood. All these oils can be potentially very harmful if ingested or used improperly.

25% Dilution. This is reccomended for those intending to use an essential oil on children 6 months to 6 yrs of age. It is recommended that you refrain from using essential oils on children under the age of 2, unless approved by your healthcare provider.
25% - 1 drop per 4 teaspoons of carrier oil.

1% Dilution. This percentage is recommended for children over 6 yrs, pregnant women, elderly adults, people who have sensitive skin issues, and those with preexisting conditions. This is the dilution recommended when using essential oils topically, for massage, or when adding to in lotions and rubs.

1% - 1 drop per teaspoon of carrier oil or 3-6 drops per ounce.

2% Dilution. Ideal for most healthy adults. For the use in aromatherapy or topical application.

2% - 2 drops per teaspoon of carrier oil or 5-12 drops per ounce

3% Dilution. Ideal for treating temporary health problems. Topical application for muscle discomfort, injury or respiratory problems.

3% - 3 drops per teaspoon of carrier oil or 10-18 drops per ounce

25% Dilution. There are several essential oils suitable to be used at this strength. Several can be used with little or no dilution. This dilution percentage is recommended for healthy adults, yet caution should still be considered as some may notice irritation or increased sensitivity to oils.

25% dilution - 25 drops per teaspoon of carrier oil or 120-150 drops per ounce.

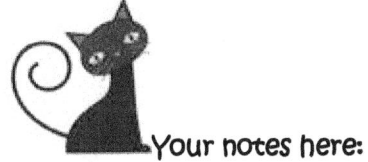Your notes here:

How Many Drops of Essential Oils Should I Put in My Diffuser?

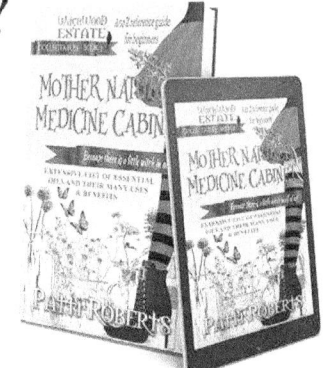

Diffuser Size	Number of Drops
100ml	3-5
200ml	6-10
300ml	9-12
400ml	12-15
500ml	15-20

LIST OF ESSENTIAL OILS –BENEFITS & USES.

Sourced from various plant and flowers using a steam distillation process, essential oils are extremely concentrated.

> *There are hundreds of varieties of essential oils available on the market today, each with their own unique properties and uses. Wellness, prevention, healing, treatment, cleaning, and spiritual advancement.*

There are many ways one can obtain the health benefits from these oils:

- Direct inhalation.
- Orally.
- Topically.
- Diffuser.
- Spray.

This book for beginners features some of the most popular essential oils available and will show you how to start!

This book belongs to

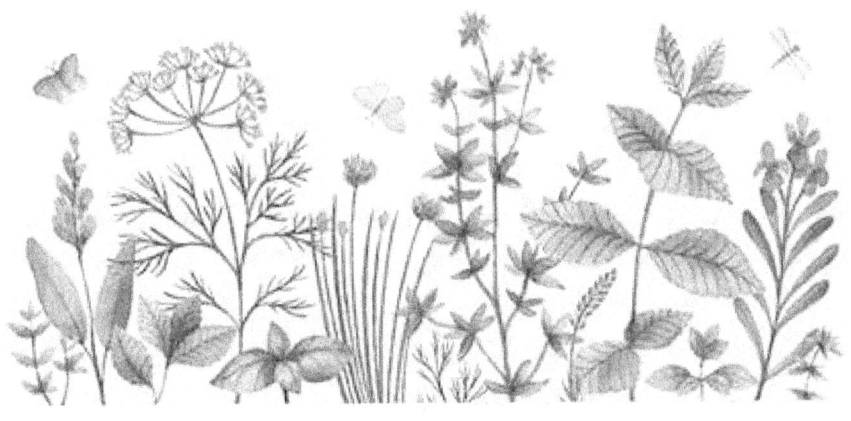

ALLSPICE

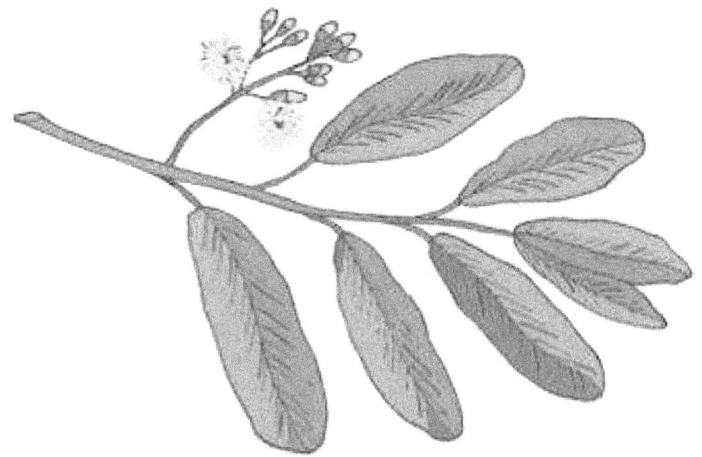

When applied, allspice has a numbing, anesthetic effect. Only locally effective, it does not affect the central nervous system. This can help endure certain discomforts such as, neuralgia, bone and muscular injuries, joint strain, as well as pains from insect bites and stings.

Anesthetic, analgesic, antiseptic, antioxidant, relaxant, stimulant, and a tonic. It relieves pain and relaxes the body and mind. Masculine. It is used in the preparation of perfumes, candles, and cosmetics.

Blends well with: Bergamot, wild orange, vanilla, clove, cinnamon, lavender, ylang ylang and citrus oils; lemon, lime, and grapefruit.

Diffuser: Diffusing the oil around your home or office is a great tonic for the mind. It can help relieve stresses and anxiety by calming the nerves and uplifting the spirit.

Add 5 drops to your diffuser. Diffusing allspice essential oil at night may help will help you sleep better by relieving anxiety - a common condition in people with sleep complaints.

Massage: Ideal for massage, arthritic and muscular applications.
1 drop per ½ tbsp. of carrier oil to relieve joint pain.

Beauty: To make your own exfoliate, mix 2 drops each of allspice and lavender with ½ cup of sugar and ½ cup of coconut oil. Don't forget your heels!

Health: Before applying allspice essential oil to your skin, dilute it with a suitable carrier oils like coconut oil, olive oil, or jojoba.

People suffering from rheumatism or arthritis may find relief from rubbing this oil into their joints. It will also help relieve joint and muscle pain after a long day on your feet or exercise.

Applying allspice essential oil on your temples may relieve a headache or sinus congestion.

Apply diluted allspice oil to insect bites or stings to soothe the pain. Along with its its analgesic properties, allspice has antiseptic properties which protect against infection. Ideal for cleaning wounds and preventing the growth of bad bacteria.

For congestion, add a few drops of the oil to a bowl of hot water. Lean over the bowl with your head covered by a towel while inhaling the vapors for as long as needed.

ANGELICA

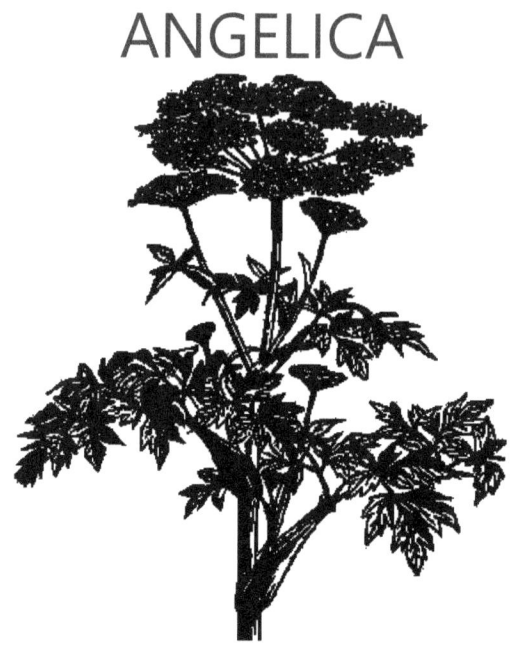

Angelica comes from the Greek word "angelos" meaning "messenger." Protection against negative energy.

Anti-spasmodic, carminative, depurative, digestive, diuretic, hepatic, and stimulates blood flow in the pelvic areas. Expectorant, nervine, stimulant, stomachic, and a tonic. Calms spasms, reduces flatulence, purifies the blood, promotes perspiration, improves in digestion, increases urination, and aids in removing toxins from the body. Angelica oil is also good for liver and stomach, relieves blocked menstruation, expels phlegm, reduces a fever, cures nervous disorders, and tones the body. Alleviates feelings of hopelessness, as well as fatigue and stress-related disorders.

Blends well with; Basil, geranium, grapefruit, lavender, chamomile, lemon, mandarin, and patchouli.

How to use.

Diffuse: Angelica essential oil can promote feelings of peace as well as helping to eradicate general feelings of negativity and anxiety. It has a musky and earthy aroma. Add 3 drops to your diffuser.

Massage: add a few drops of angelica to a carrier oil for a soothing massage oil to aid in digestion and improve circulation.

Beauty: Add 2 drops of angelica, 2 drops of frankincense, 2 drops of rosehip oil to a Tbsp. of coconut oil and gently apply.

Health: Breathe easy recipe. Add 1 drop Angelica, 4 drops spruce, 2 drops orange, 2 drops clary sage, 4 drops of eucalyptus, 3 drops of peppermint for a general breath assisting diffuser blend.

Add ingredients to your bathwater for a calming soak.

For menstrual problems, dilute your oil with a carrier oil and massage into the abdomen at bedtime. You can also add a few drops to a warm compress and apply it to your stomach.

> *Angelica essential oil is an effective remedy for sinus problems or migraines. Massage a few drops into your temples, or inhale it directly from the bottle, cloth, orhands.*

ARBORVITAE "THE TREE OF LIFE."

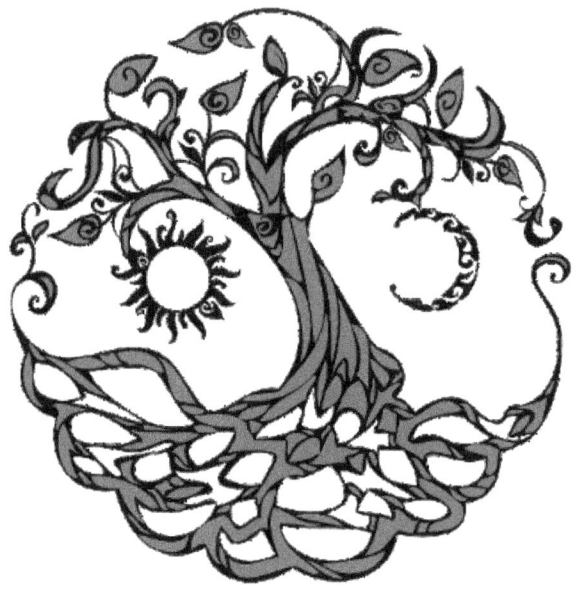

In modern times, popularity for this wonderful essential oil with its bounty of natural benefits, has grown.

This bright orange essential oil boasts a variety of uses. It is a natural cleansing agent, a powerful bug repellent, and it has been known to help promote a naturally healthy skin. It also preserves wood.

Blends well with; Birch, Cedarwood, Cassia, and Eucalyptus essential oil.

> **Diffuse:** *Add 3-4 drops to your diffuser to create an air freshener to fight airborne bacteria and to repel insects inside the home. Promotes a calming, tranquil feeling.*

Massage: Can be used directly on the skin in large doses with caution (use carrier oil if you have sensitive skin). For Respiratory support, massage 1 drop on the throat and chest every few hours for relief.

Beauty: Apply 1–2 drops to problem areas on the skin. For facial cleansers and moisturizers - amazing benefits on skin health and tone. Can be applied directly to the skin in small doses or mix with a moisturizer or lotions. Arborvitae penetrates deep into pores, delivering moisture to your skin. It's also a natural cleansing agent.

Health: Dab Arborvitae on wrists and ankles for a natural way of repelling insects to avoid toxic commercially produced repellants.

Household: Add 8 drops to a spray bottle with water, then spray on surfaces. Repels all sorts of insects, including moths and mosquitos. Add drops to wooden coat hangers or inside drawers to deter moths and silverfish. Add to your bucket to clean and polish wooden floors.

Add your notes here:

BASIL

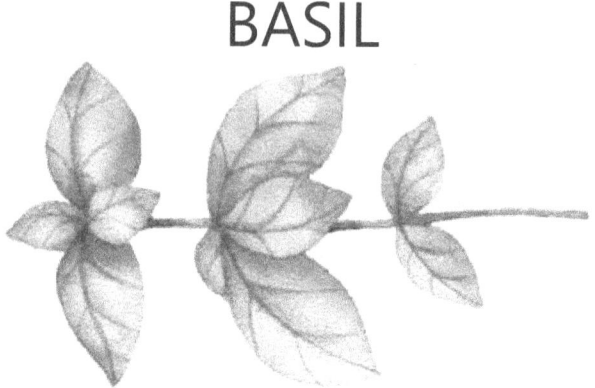

Basil oil has become very popular due to its high linalool content. Its rich and soothing aroma makes it great for relieving stress.

Carminative, anti-spasmodic, analgesic, anti-bacterial, and ophthalmic (relating to or resembling the eye). Skin care, indigestion, infections, respiratory problems, stress disorders, circulation issues, discomfort, and vomiting. While this oil is far less reactive than some other oils, it can cause skin irritation on those who have sensitive skin or those who have adverse reactions to concentrated substances.

Blends well with; Bergamot oil, black pepper oil, cedarwood, fennel oil, ginger oil, geranium, grapefruit, lavender, lemon, marjoram, and neroli oil.

How to use.

Diffuse: Inhaling basil oil can help to restore alertness and fight fatigue. Add 3-4 drops to a diffuser. Ideal for studying or reading to improve focus and concentration. Increases sense of peace and calm. Minimize negative thoughts, feelings. Basil aids in eliminate odor-causing bacteria and mold from your home and furniture. Basil oil pairs nicely with citrus-based aromas; lime, lemon, and orange. Suffering from cold or flu? Add to your bathwater with a few drops of eucalyptus and lavender oil to help you relax.

Massage: Dilute Basil oil with coconut oil before applying to directly to your skin. Basil oil can sometimes cause skin reactions if you have sensitive skin, so avoid using it on your face, neck or chest until you have done a skin test. Massage into the skin to soothe aching muscles. Basil promotes a soothing, cooling feeling, and the strong aroma helps clear nostrils during colds. Rub diluted basil and coconut into painful muscles or joints.

Beauty: Add a few drops basil into a facial cleanser to reduce the appearance of skin blemishes. Soothing to the skin, basil also helps to unclog pores. Combine basil with tea tree oil in a facial cleanser to soothe and cleanse while reducing the redness and swelling of blemishes. Skin breakouts are usually caused by the built-up of bacteria and excess oil. Basil oil is there for an ideal home remedy for acne. Using a cotton ball, apply 1 - 2 drops of basil oil diluted in coconut oil to the affected area during your morning and evening cleansing routine.

Health: Fight chronic infections, including bronchitis and respiratory illnesses, by mixing basil with eucalyptus, and rosemary oil. Helps to reduce infections of the lungs and respiratory tract. Diffuse or add to a carrier oil and massage into chest and the bottom of feet. Wear socks for best results.
For a bug repellent, dilute several drops of basil oil with a carrier oil and massage into the skin or to soothe bites – use as needed.

Household: Use basil oil to remove bacteria from kitchens and bathroom surfaces, preventing contamination. Also combats mold. Spray it inside your toilet, shower and garbage cans. Add to spray bottle with water and shake before use.

BERGAMOT

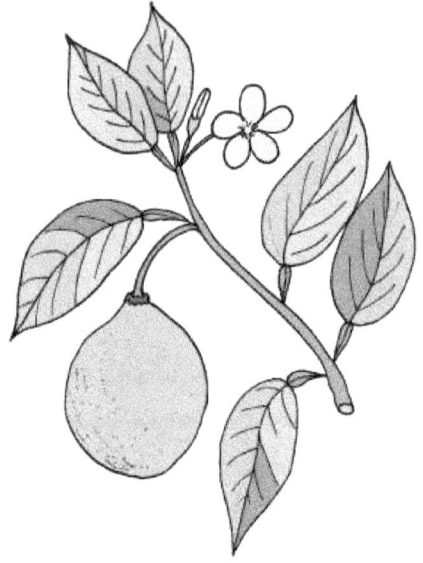

> **For the little witch in all of us:** *Used in protective rituals, bergamot also brings prosperity when a drop is placed on the palms of each hand.*

Bergamot oil is what gives Earl Grey Tea its unique taste! It has a sweet and fruity aroma with is both uplifting and relaxing.

Bergamot is helpful when dealing with dependency, such as smoking, drugs and alcohol. Emotional support, skin problems, skin purifying.

Antibiotic, antiseptic, antispasmodic, sedative, analgesic, antidepressant, disinfectant, and digestive in nature.

Reduces body odor, relieves spasms, soothes pain, improves mood, fights depression, heals cuts, and promotes healing.

Blends well with; Arborvitae, frankincense, lavender, lime, patchouli, chamomile, rose, and Ylang-Ylang. Other popular oil combinations include black pepper, cypress, frankincense, jasmine, mandarin, rosemary, sage, sandalwood, and vetiver.

> *Diffuse:* Add 3-4 drops and diffuse in the classroom, office, or home to ease stress and tension.

Massage: 1 part essential oil: 4 parts carrier oil. For the treatment of aching muscles and joints, dilute 5 drops of bergamot in a carrier oil and massage into the affected area of your body.

To relieve headaches, massage a few drops into your temples and neck or inhale it directly. Apply 1-2 drops topically to the bottom of each foot before bed at night. Alternatively, you can dilute several drops of oil with a carrier oil to use in a calming massage.

Beauty: Many women's perfumes and men's colognes contain bergamot oils. Bergamot oil is used to treat common skin conditions including ache, eczema and psoriasis. To treat skin conditions, add a few drops of bergamot to a dampened cotton ball and apply directly to the problem area daily.

Health: A powerful antifungal oil, it effectively destroys many strains of fungus including nail fungus. To treat a wound, burn or bite, apply diluted bergamot oil to the affected area as needed.

To ease a fever, diffuse bergamot essential oil night and day.

Household: Diffuse bergamot around the home to eliminate cooking or tobacco smells.

Bergamot essential oil is an effective natural repellent - keeping unwanted bugs and pests at bay, including mosquitoes, ants, and silverfish. Add to your diffuser or a spray bottle. Add drops to wooden coat hangers or drawers to protect your clothing from insects.

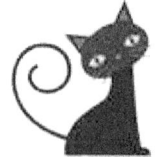 Add your own recipes and tips here:

Sunlight is more powerful than any drug; it is safe, effective, and available free of charge. If it could be patented, it would be hyped as the greatest medical breakthrough in history. It's that good. ~ Mike Adams, natural health researcher and author.

BLACK PEPPER

Never apply black pepper near the eyes, in the ears, or near any other sensitive area.

Digestive, antispasmodic, antirheumatic, antiarthritic, antibacterial, carminative, and an antioxidant. Aids in digestion and increases perspiration. Helps remove toxins. Remove gases from the intestines, soothes spasms, and helps to treat arthritis and rheumatism. Removes toxins from the body. Inhibits bacterial growth and neutralizes free radicals. Stimulates circulation, promotes emotional balance. Stimulates an appetite and reduces cholesterol levels.

Blends well with; Lavender, sandalwood, clove, sage, lemon, lime, mandarin, grapefruit, bergamot, clary sage, clove, ylang ylang, ginger, coriander, frankincense, and fennel.

Diffuse: Place 3 - 4 drops of oil in your diffuser. Its spicy and warm aroma is stimulating and empowering.

> *Diffusing black pepper oil help you remain sharp and focused. To reduce your cigarette cravings, diffuse black pepper oil or inhale it directly from the bottle during cravings. Helps ease anxiety and nervousness.*

Compress: Mix about 10 drops of black pepper essential oil and about four ounces of warm water in a basin. Soak a cloth into mixture and apply the compress to the affected area. Hold the compress to the area for a few minutes and reapply as necessary.

Massage: 1 part essential oil to 1 part vegetable oil. Add to a carrier oil like coconut oil, jojoba oil, or almond oil. Ideal for a relaxing and restoring massage and applying directly to overworked muscles.

Health: Black pepper oil suppresses cigarette withdrawal symptoms and lowers blood pressure. Black pepper oil can be safely inhaled directly from the bottle.

> *To help detoxify the body, apply 2 - 3 drops to the bottoms of the feet and put on a pair of socks. Also warms a chilled body and gives you a boost of energy as well.*

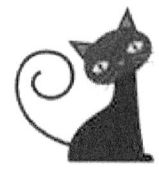 **Add your own recipes and tips here:**

CANNABIS

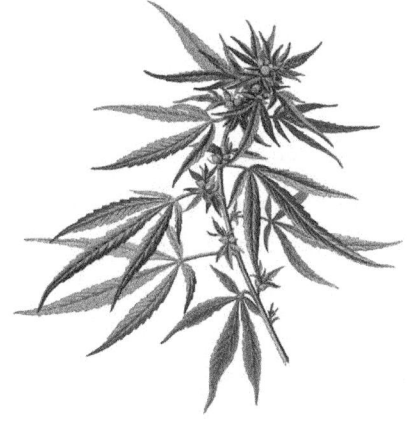

"A weed is a plant whose virtue is not yet known." ~Ralph Waldo Emerson

Cannabis is derived from the cannabis sativa plant. Used by ancient civilizations for Tantric rituals and spiritual meditation, cannabis essential oil's therapeutic aroma enhances emotional and mental well-being by releasing stress and relaxing the body while lifting the spirit. Cannabis contain high amounts of a substance commonly referred to as THC - or tetrahydrocannabinol - which is well known for its psychotropic abilities. This oil treats a wide range of illnesses including cancer, anorexia, pain, and inflammation. Improves the quality of sleep, boosts appetite, optimizes digestion, reduces pain, and protects heart health.

There is much more to learn about the healing qualities of this oil. It has also been used for a number of neurodegenerative disorders such as Alzheimer's disease, Parkinson's and Tourette's syndrome. Cannabis and hemp oil come from the same species – cannabis sativa. Hemp oil, however, is quite different to cannabis oil. Hemp is commonly used for topical ointments, fiber and paper.

Cannabis treatments are effective in reducing anxiety in those suffering from PTSD.

Blends well with; Eucalyptus bergamot, lemon, lime, orange, and lavender essential oil.

Beauty: Add a couple of drops of cannabis to a carrier oil to promote a healthy-looking skin. When applied topically, cannabis oil stimulates the shedding of dead skin cells and promotes the growth of new ones. Add a few drops to your bath water for a relaxing bath at the end of the day.

Health: Cannabis oil slows the signs of aging and reduces skin spots due to its natural antioxidants that fight against cellular damage caused by free radicals. Cannabis essential oil is an effective treatment method for psoriasis and eczema.

Tests have shown the ability of cannabis oil to treat eye conditions such as glaucoma and macular degeneration. Glaucoma is a serious optic nerve disease that can lead to blindness. So not apply cannabis essential oil directly to the eye, but rather through aromatherapy.

Lifestyle and Diet Changes:

When using cannabis oil treatment for cancer, steps must be taken in changing your diet, and lifestyle. Studies show that cancer cannot sustain in an alkaline body. You will need to eat an alkaline diet comprising of lots of organic greens every day. Plant protein fights the growth of cancer. Start drinking as many raw fruits and vegetable smoothies as much as possible. You may like to check out the next book in the series, "Little Book Of Smoothies," for some great blending ideas.

Eat little to no meat or dairy products, the proteins in these foods will promote cancer growth. You should also stop eating sugar. Replace the use of sugar with natural alternative like dates or raw honey.

Let us hope that further studies will continue to prove the health benefits derived from cannabis oil – which in most cases, is a healthier alternative to the side effects of pharmaceutical drugs.

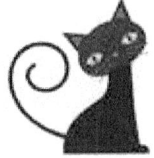 **Add your own recipes and tips here:**

> *This is like the Holy Grail of cancer medicine; vitamin D produced a drop in cancer rates greater than that for quitting smoking, or indeed any other countermeasure in existence. ~ Dennis Mangan, clinical laboratory scientist.*

CARDAMOM

Mix cardamom with rose and sandalwood for a sensual perfume.

Spicy, with sweet, floral undertones, woody. Soothing and calming, the oil has a cool and minty flavor, so it pairs well with the tastes of smoothies, salads, and meats. Anti-spasmodic, neutralizes the negative effects of chemotherapy, reduces nausea.

Protects wounds and incisions, increases libido, promote digestion, and maintains optimal stomach health. Increases urination by removing extra salt, bile, water, toxins and fat from the body.

Blends well with; Rose oil, bergamot oil, orange, cedarwood, and spice oils such as black pepper, cinnamon oil, clove oil, and ginger oil.

How to use.
Diffuse: Add 4 drops to a diffuser to increase a positive mood and clear the mind. Diffusing and inhaling will also make a person feel happier.

Combine with lavender and clove to relieve stress or overwhelming feelings. This combination can also help turn around a bad mood.

Massage: To relieve stress from external areas of the body, mix a couple of drops with a carrier oil and apply to the desired area. The fragrant scent will improve your mental state as it is massaged into the skin. Apply to the chest to help alleviate congested breathing.

Combine with peppermint, spearmint, and ginger to relieve aching muscles or difficulty with breathing. Apply it to any sore area to relieve pain.

Cardamom oil in a carrier oils such as almond works as a sensual massage oil.

Romance Blend: 2 drops cardamom, 4 drops jasmine oil, 4 drops sandalwood, 2 drops rose oil in a 15 ml with your favorite carrier oil.

Beauty: Mix cardamom with rose and sandalwood for a sensual perfume.

Health: Add 5 drops of cardamom to water and gargle. Cardamom oil disinfects and eliminates bad breath. Cardamom oil can help cure erectile dysfunctions, impotence, loss of libido, and frigidity.

Soothe a tummy: 4 drops cardamom, 5 drops angelica oil, 5 drops clary sage oil, 5 drops chamomile oil in 2 Tbsp of your choice of carrier oil.

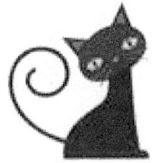 **Add your own recipes and tips here:**

CASSIA

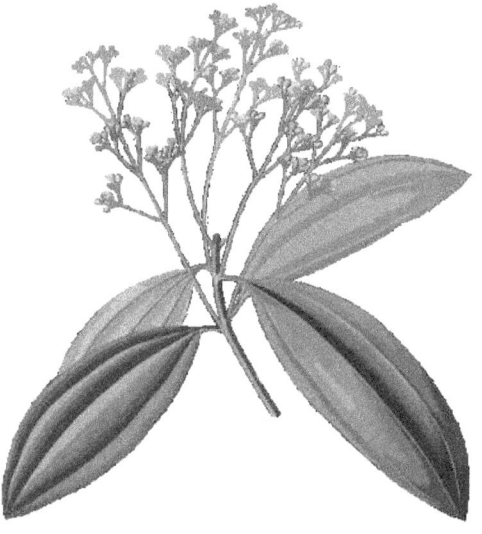

The woody, spiciness, generates a sense of well-being. Sexual stimulant, improves digestion.

Anti-diarrheal, antidepressant, antiviral, antimicrobial, antirheumatic and an anti-arthritic. Astringent, circulatory, carminative, and a stimulant. Eliminate loose stool and diarrhea. Aids in depression, lifts mood. Reduces vomiting, slows milk flow, inhibit microbial growth, treats rheumatism and arthritis, tightens muscles and prevents hair loss. Reduces hemorrhaging, fights viral infections, removes excess gas, improves blood & lymphatic circulation, relieves obstructed menstruation, and reduces a fever.

Blends well with; Black pepper, chamomile, coriander, caraway, frankincense, ginger, geranium, nutmeg, and rosemary.

How to use.

Diffuse: When diffused Cassia has been known to produce feelings of arousal. When diffusing alone use 1 - 4 drops. Reduce this to 1 - 2 when in combination with other scents such as Clove, Ginger, or White Fir.

Diffuse 2 - 3 drops of cassia oil to calm your nerves.

> *Combine with Clove and Ginger during the holiday season to evoke the smell of grandma's house.*

To treat cold and flu; diffuse 2–3 drops of cassia oil.

Massage: Combine a drop or 2 with a carrier oil for a warming massage to relieve achy joints and sore muscles.

Beauty: Cassia oil strengthens gums and hair, tightens muscles and lifts the skin.

Health: Cassia oil inhibits the microbial growth and prevents diarrhea from occurring due to its fiber content and resulting in healthy bowel movements.

Cassia oil fights depression, uplifts mood, and induces positive feelings in the body and mind.

Cassia essential oil improves circulation and creates a warming feeling to the joints and other parts of the body affected by rheumatism and arthritis.

Cassia relaxes menstrual cramps.

Offers relief from symptoms such as headaches, nausea.

Cassia oil has shown to naturally treat type 2 diabetes by lowering blood sugar levels.

For digestive health add 2–3 drops of cassia oil with equal parts of a carrier oil such as coconut or jojoba oil and rub on your feet or abdomen.

To kill a fungal infection, add 1–2 drops of cassia oil with equal parts of a carrier oil and rub on the affected area twice daily.

To uplift your mood and 4 - 5 drops of cassia oil to a warm bath.

To treat nausea place 4–5 drops of cassia oil on a handkerchief and inhale whenever you are feeling nauseous.

Household: Cassia oil has substantial cleansing properties and when combined with water and white vinegar can make an aromatic and effective surface cleaner.

Cassia oil is an effective mosquito repellant and works as an all-natural and chemical-free remedy. Add 2 – 3 drops of carrier oil and massage into skin.

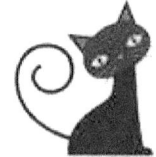 **Add your own recipes and tips here:**

We estimate that vitamin D deficiency is the most common medical condition in the world. ~ Dr. Michael F. Holick, Vitamin D expert.

CEDARWOOD

Cedarwood essential oil is widely used to improve sleep quality, promote healthy skin, repel insects, and create a beautiful aroma. Antispasmodic, tonic, astringent, diuretic, expectorant, insecticidal, antiseptic, sedative, and a fungicide. Heals wounds. Increase urination, removal of toxins, water, salt and fat from the body. Regulates menstrual cycles, cures coughs and colds. Reduces inflammation and nervous disturbances and inhibits fungal growth and infections.

Blends well with; Bergamot, benzoin, cypress, cinnamon, frankincense, juniper, jasmine, lemon, lime, lavender, rose, neroli, rosemary, juniper, basil, thyme, clary sage, cypress, eucalyptus, lime, neroli, vetiver, and sandalwood.

Diffuse: Add 3-4 drops to a diffuser to increase feelings of comfort, vitality, and wellness.

Consider adding 2 drops of bergamot, lavender, or chamomile oils to induce a greater state of relaxation.

> *To help you focus, diffuse 2 drops of cedarwood, 2 drops of vetiver, and 2drops of lavender.*

Massage: Dilute several drops with a carrier oil and massage into the skin to reduce muscle and joint inflammation. Also works as a topical antiseptic.

Mix cedarwood essential oil with coconut oil and rub the mixture into your body to help with wounds, scars or infections.

Beauty: Add 1-2 drops to coconut oil to enhance skin clarity and smoothness.

Cedarwood oil can stimulate the hair follicles and increase circulation to the scalp. Massage the oil into your scalp. Wait for 30 minutes before rinsing. Add several drops to shampoo or conditioner bottles to add shine.

Make your own face scrub by mixing 7 drops of cedarwood essential oil and blending with a tablespoon of Epsom salt and a tablespoon of coconut oil. Mix the ingredients together until you get a paste. Use the blend to exfoliate your face to help cleans the skin and eliminate acne.

Health: Cedarwood essential oil prevents wounds from turning septic. It can be applied externally to wounds as an antiseptic.

Cedarwood oil helps soothes toothaches, strengthens gums, and protects teeth from falling out.

2 – 3 drops of cedarwood in a diffuser will promote a good night's sleep when suffering from a cough and cold.

For arthritis, make yourself a warm bath with 5 - 10 drops of cedarwood essential oil.

Cedarwood is often used by those suffering from insomnia.

Household: When used in diffusers, cedarwood deters mosquitoes, flies, and other insects. Sprinkled on pillows or sheets at night to ward off mosquitoes and other bugs while you sleep.

To create a multi-oil natural insect repellant, consider adding drops of basil and thyme. Oils such as cinnamon or bergamot will add a spicy or sweet note to the repellant.

> *Add several drops to a cotton ball or on wooden coat hangers and place in a closet to deter the presence of moths. Also ideal for areas like drawers and linen cupboards.*

Spray diluted cedarwood essential oil with water on your bed lined and soft furnishing to keep pests away.

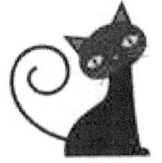 **Add your own recipes and tips here:**

> *"If people let the government decide what foods they eat and what medicines they take, their bodies will soon be in as sorry a state as are the souls who live under tyranny."- Thomas Jefferson*

CHAMOMILE

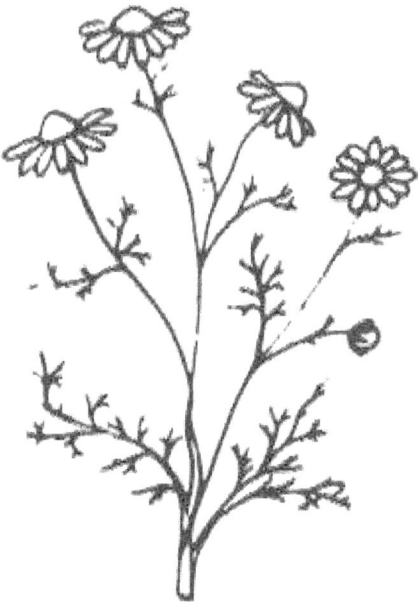

There are two plants known as chamomile: the more popular German chamomile (Matricaria recutita) and Roman, or English, chamomile (Chamaemelum nobile). Although belonging to different plant species, they are both used to treat the same health problems.

> *Next to lavender, Roman or English chamomile is found in many homes because of its many qualities.*

Sweet, woody; apple, peach. Anti-spasmodic, antidepressant, anti-neuralgic, antiseptic, antibiotic, carminative, cholagogue, cicatrisant, analgesic, hepatic, nervine, digestive, tonic, bactericidal, anti-inflammatory, and anti-infectious. Soothes spasms, protects wounds from becoming septic and infected, curbs biotic growth and infections. Fights depression and uplift moods. Cures neuralgic pain by reducing swelling in the effected vessels and soothes inflammation. Eliminates gases, promotes discharge and reduces fever. Chamomile is one of the most popular and useful essential oils.

Blends well with; Ginger, geranium, lavender, rose, ylang-ylang, bergamot, lemon, neroli oil, clary sage, and patchouli oil.

How to use.

Diffuse: To fight anxiety and feelings of depression, diffuse 5 drops or inhale the oil directly from the bottle.

For a restful night's sleep, diffuse chamomile oil next to your bed.

Try combining Chamomile, ginger, peppermint and lavender oil and diffuse.

Winter Relief: diffuse 2 drop spearmint oil, 2 drops Roman chamomile, 2 drops lavender oil.

Massage: 3 drops chamomile, 3 drops helichrysum oil, 2 drops birch oil in ½ oz carrier oil and applied topically as needed.

Beauty: Roman chamomile promotes a smooth, healthy skin. To treat skin conditions and slow the signs of aging, add 2–3 drops to cotton ball and apply to the problem area. If you have sensitive skin, dilute chamomile with a carrier oil before applying it topically.

Health: When applied topically, Roman chamomile oil helps relieve skin irritations that may be due to food sensitivities.

To calm children, diffuse chamomile oil or dilute 1–2 drops with coconut oil and apply the mixture topically to the temples, stomach, wrists, back of neck and the bottoms of feet.

To promote heart health, apply 2–4 drops topically over the heart.

Add 6 drops to your bath before bed to induce a calm and restful sleep.

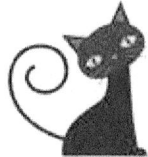 Add your own recipes and tips here:

"The person who takes medicine must recover twice, once from the disease and once from the medicine." - William Osler, M.D. -

CILANTRO / CORIANDER

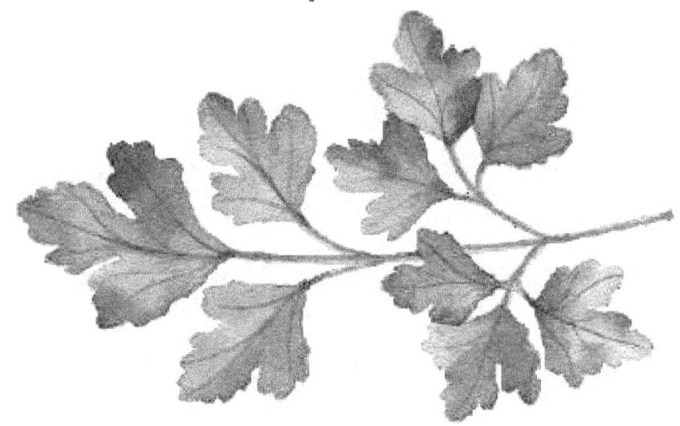

For the little witch in love: *A love oil used to anoint candles.*

Bright, crisp, fresh, sweet. Cilantro oil improves appetite, cures nausea, and can eliminate vomiting as a symptom.

Improves digestion, supports healthy skin, antioxidant. Rich in antioxidants. Cleanser and detoxifier. Soothing to the skin.

Blends well with; Bergamot, Cinnamon, Grapefruit, Ginger, Neroli, Lemon, Lime, Orange, other Citrus oils, and spearmint.

Diffuse: Diffused, this essential oil will relieve stress and calm mind. Also aids with restful sleep and general relaxation.

Mixed with other oils, a few drops of cilantro in a diffuser creates a wonderful aroma.

Massage: Cilantro oil can be combined with a carrier oil and massaged into sore areas.

Health: Are you ready for some fun in the bedroom? Cilantro essential oil arouses the libido, as well as cures temporary impotency, erectile dysfunctions, and general loss of interest in sex.

Cilantro essential oil cleans the blood of toxins, and acts as a detoxifier. It helps to remove regular toxins like uric acid, heavy metals, and hormones produced by the body.

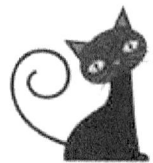 **Add your own recipes and tips here:**

"This large and expensive stock of drugs will be unnecessary....The common resources of the lancet, a garden, a kitchen, fresh air, cool water, exercise, will be sufficient to cure all the diseases that are at present under the power of medicine." - Dr. Benjamin Rush.

CINNAMON

For the magical witch. A high-vibration oil, cinnamon is used for personal protection. Mixed with sandalwood, it creates an aroma for magic. Ideal for meditation and illumination.

Reminiscent of a freshly baked apple pies. Spicy, woody, camphorous.

Antibacterial, antifungal, anti-microbial, astringent, anti-clotting, stimulating, cooling, and carminative. Respiratory problems, skin infections, blood circulation issues, infections, wound healing, pain relief, menstruation problems, breastfeeding, heart disorders, diabetes, colon cancer, indigestion, and relief for bad breath!

Blends well with; basil, clove, eucalyptus, fennel, ginger, marjoram, orange, mandarin, vetiver, agarwood, lemon, rosemary, geranium, lavender, cardamom, and cedarwood.

Diffuse: Diffused cinnamon to create a sensual atmosphere. Add ginger, cedarwood, and vetiver for an exotic, stimulating blend. A diffusion of cinnamon can energize a sluggish mind.

Diffuse a combination of 2 drops cinnamon, 3 drops mandarin oil, and 3 drops orange to lift spirits.

> *Diffuse Cinnamon oil to prevent fatigue, moodiness, sugar cravings, and overeating. Try adding a couple of drops to your chest, wrists, and clothes.*

Massage: 1 drop of cinnamon in 0.5 oz carrier oil and massage into legs, arms and joints to warm and relax the body.

3 drops clove, 3 drops lemon essential oil, 2 drops cinnamon, 1 drop rosemary essential oil, and 1 drop eucalyptus essential oil in ½ oz of carrier oil. Apply to bottoms of your feet then put on a pair of socks.

Health: Cinnamon helps in regulating insulin release, keeping blood sugar stable and preventing chronic fatigue, moodiness, and sugar cravings.

For treating skin conditions – such as rashes and acne, combine cinnamon oil to coconut oil and apply to the skin to take advantage of its antimicrobial benefits.

Household: Deodorizing Room Spray: 2 drop cinnamon, 3 drops clove, 3 drops cedarwood oil, 6 drops tea tree oil, 6 drops lemon oil. Mix with 2 cups of water and use in a spray bottle.

CLARY SAGE

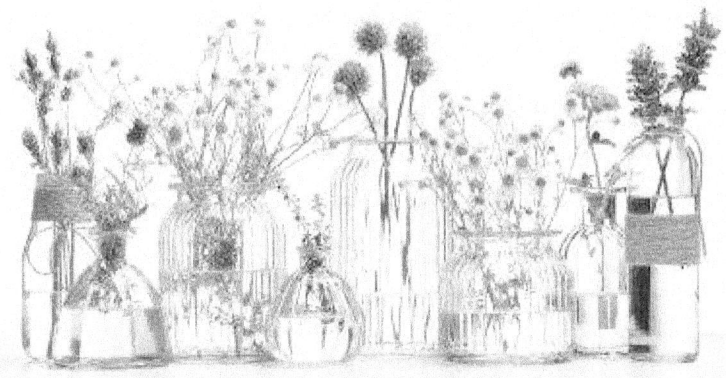

Fresh, floral, dry, sweet herbaceous, tea-like. Long considered "woman's oil," clary sage's benefits is in its calming influence on the body and mind. It also supports emotional and feminine functions. Clary sage serves as an antidepressant and is one of the best natural remedies for anxiety.

Clary sage essential oil can substitute many of over-the-counter products. Instead of investing in expensive lotions, apply clary sage oil to irritated skin. It should help soothe any itching or burning. Irritated skin can also be remedied by adding a few drops to your warm bath water. Massage into the abdomen to relieve menstrual cramps.

Antidepressant, antiseptic, aphrodisiac, astringent, bactericidal, antispasmodic, carminative, deodorant, digestive, euphoric, hypotensive, nervine, sedative, and improves memory. Fights depression and uplifts mood, soothes spasms, protects wound from becoming septic. Reduces sexual dysfunction and increases libido, causes contractions, kills bacteria and slows bacterial growth. Removes excess gas, eliminates body odor, improves digestion, relieves menstruation, lowers blood pressure. Improves the health of the nervous system.

Blends well with; Citrus oils along with bergamot lavender, cypress, frankincense, geranium, rose, vetiver, jasmine, juniper oil, neroli oil, cedarwood oil, black pepper, coriander, grapefruit, chamomile, orange, lemon, rose, and sandalwood oil.

Diffuse: Adding a few drops of clary sage to your diffuser will help in reducing anxious moods by creating a calming atmosphere. This is useful after a long, busy day at work, or if you need to focus on a particular task. Eases stress, depression and insomnia.

For stress relief, diffuse 2–3 drops of clary sage essential oil. You can also add 2 drops of lavender oil.

For relaxation, diffuse 6 drops of clary sage oil with 2 drops of frankincense, and 2 drops of orange.

Mood Balancing: 6 drops bergamot oil, 6 drops clary sage oil, 2 drops jasmine oil.

Massage: To soothe cramps and pains, combine 6 drops of clary sage with a teaspoon of carrier oil like jojoba or coconut oil.

To ease digestion, try a hot compress with 4–6 drops of clary sage oil.

Massage tired feet with clary sage and coconut oil.

Beauty: Combine 5 drops of clary sage oil with a teaspoon of jojoba or coconut oil for a perfect skin moisturizer.

If your hair is dull or damaged, combine a few drops of clary sage to your conditioner, and apply to scalp to promote a healthy head of hair. Your hair will become smooth and shiny.

Health: Clary sage's many benefits have been used for cramps, uncomfortable menstrual cycles, hot flashes and hormonal imbalances. Well known for increaseing circulation, supporting the digestive system, and improveing eye health.

To relieve asthma symptoms, mix 5 drops of clary sage oil with 2 drops of lavender oil in a carrier oil and massage on the chest or back.

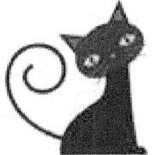 Add your own recipes and tips here:

"The introduction of homeopathy forced the old school doctor to stir around and learn something of a rational nature about his business. You may honestly feel grateful that homeopathy survived the attempts of allopaths (the orthodox physicians to destroy it."---- Mark Twain

CLOVE

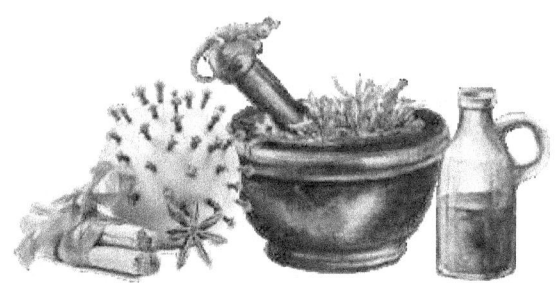

> *For the single witch: weaar to attract lovers. Inhaled, the oil incrases memory and insight.*

Clove oil is very strong and needs to be used in a diluted form. For those with sensitive skin, use sparingly. Warm, spicy, earthy, woody and musky. Clove oil is useful for boosting the immune system. Clove oil has antiviral properties which purifies the blood and increases resistance to a number of diseases. Cures infections, skin conditions, stress, headaches, respiratory problems, earaches, indigestion, nausea, blood circulation, diabetes, immune system, premature ejaculation, cholera, and sties. Also aids in the treatment of insect bites and stings.

Blends well with: Basil essential oil, rosemary essential oil, rose oil, cinnamon essential oil, grapefruit essential oil, lemon oil, nutmeg oil, peppermint essential oil, orange essential oil, lavender oil, clary sage, frankincense oil, sandalwood, ylang-ylang, and geranium essential oil.

> **Diffuse:** *If you are feeling tired and need a pick-me-up, add 3 - 4 drops of clove essential oil to a diffuser. It can also be combined with other energizing essential oils.*

Combine 2 drops of clove with 4 drops of orange, 3 drops of lemon, and 3 drops of grapefruit, and diffuse. This would be a great to start the day.

To relieve lung discomfort, diffuse a combination of 3 drops clove oil, 5 drops lavender with 3 drops of clary sage for relief.

Clove oil repels insects. Add 4 - 5 drops to your diffuser and leave outside to deter mosquitos before hosting your barbeque.

Beauty: Mix a few drops of clove oil with organic honey or another carrier oil and apply mixture to the skin. This can help to heal wounds and clear up blemishes.

Health: Clove oil helps control blood sugar levels, making it useful to patients suffering with diabetes.

Toothache: Add a few drops of clove oil to a cotton ball and press against the problem tooth. This will numb the tooth within moments.

Before bed, gargle four ounces of water with one drop of clove oil. You can also add a drop to your toothpaste before brushing your teeth.

Household: Clove oil is commonly used in bug repellent.

Adding a few drops of clove oil on bedsheets at night will keep bugs away.

CUMIN

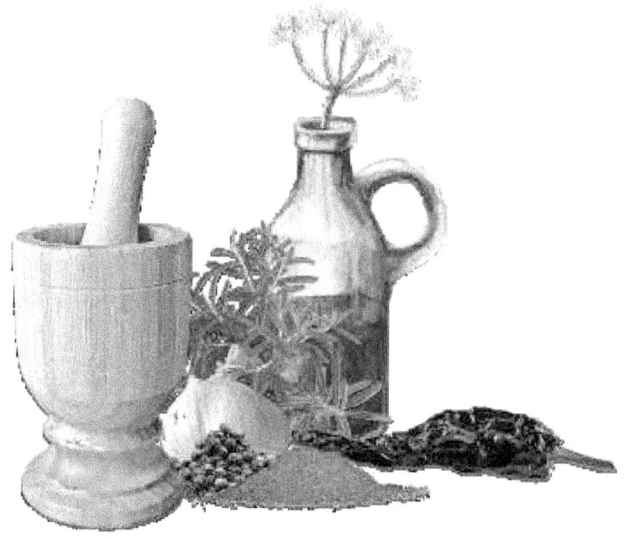

> *For the peaceful witch:* Bring peace and harmony to your home with cumin. Anoint doorways on a Friday just before sunrise while the household still sleeps.

Cumin essential oil is used in the treatment of diarrhea and cholera. Nutty and spicy. Purifying and improves digestion.

Bactericidal, carminative, antispasmodic, detoxifying, digestive, diuretic, antiseptic, stimulant, nervine. Kills bacteria and inhibits infection. Removes excess gas from the intestine, promotes digestion, increases urination, and protects wounds from becoming septic. Reduces spasms, removes toxins from the blood, regulates the menstrual cycle.

Blends well with: Angelica, Caraway, cinnamon, peppermint oil, angelica, caraway, chamomile, and Coriander.

> *Diffuse: Diffusing cumin reduces the negative emotional effects of stress.*

Diffuse to stimulate appetites before serving dinner. Use 3-4 drops.

Massage: Add 1-2 drops to a carrier oil such as avocado or coconut oil and massage into the skin to create a warming sensation.

Dilute 1 – 2 drops in a carrier oil and massage into muscles to reduce aches and pains after a workout.

Beauty: Combine 1-2 drops in carrier oil and apply to the skin to improve your complexion. Reduces the appearance of wrinkles and acne.

Add 1-2 drops to a carrier oil and apply topically to reduce the appearance of cellulite.

Health: Add a couple of drops to a carrier oil such as avocado or coconut oil. Apply to wounds as an antiseptic to stimulate healing.

For a fresh, antiseptic mouth rinse, add 1 drop to half a glass of water and gargle morning and night.

> *"If this country is to survive, the best-fed-nation myth had better be recognized for what it is: propaganda designed to produce wealth but not health" ~ Adelle Davis*

CYPRESS

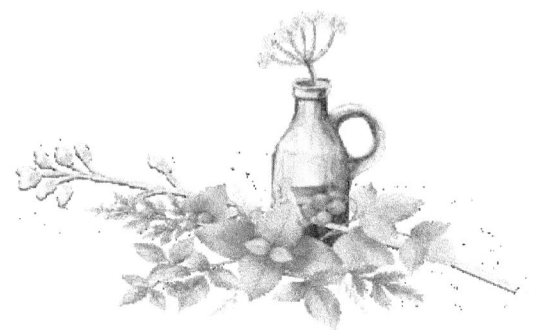

> **The earthy elemenalt witch:** *An essential oil for blessings and protection. Cypress represents the earth element. When attending the funeral of a friend, wear cypress oil to recognize that death is the doorway to another life. Wear on Samhain in memory of those who have passed on.*

Cypress essential oil is a fresh, spicy fragrance. Elevates the spirits and stimulates happiness, focus, and energy. This essential oil is valued for its capability to fight infections. Aids the respiratory system and removes toxins from the body. It also works as a stimulate, relieving stress and anxiety.

Skin health and relieves muscle soreness. Astringent, antiseptic, anti-spasmodic, deodorant, diuretic, respiratory tonic, and sedative. Removes body odor, increases urination, promotes perspiration, and soothes inflammation.

Blends well with: Lavender, vetiver, grapefruit, rose, geranium, chamomile, pine, juniper; clary sage, ylang-ylang, helichrysum, bergamot, lemon, and cedar.

Diffuse: Diffuse during times of transition or loss. Decreases feelings of anxiety. Assists in stabilizing emotions. For the mind, cypress is known to have a refreshing, cleansing effect which can dispel stress. Diffuse 5 drops of cypress oil to freshen the air.

Cypress is a useful essential oil for promoting concentration and productivity.

Diffuse 3 drops of cypress oil with 4 drops of lavender to soothe the nervous system.

For an uplifting, stress-free scent to lift feelings of joy and happiness, blend 6 drops cypress, 6 drops lavender, 3 drops vetiver, 3 drops grapefruit, and 2 drops cedar.

Massage: Blend 6 drops cypress with 5 drops rose, 2 drops geranium, and 3 drops chamomile in 2 Tbsp. of coconut or jojoba oil for a facial massage oil.

> *Blend 7 drops of Cyprus with 5 drops of lavender and 3 drops of peppermint in 2 tablespoons of coconut oil for a relaxing neck, shoulders, arms, and foot massage.*

Beauty: The antibacterial and antiseptic properties of cypress oil reduces the need for overpriced acne fighters, and pore minimizers.

Blend 5 drops cypress oil with 6 drops grapefruit, and 4 drops patchouli in a cup of sea salts with ½ cup jojoba for a detoxing salt scrub.

Cyprus oil's ability to stimulate blood flow, makes it ideal for a varicose veins homemade remedy. Add 7 drops of cypress oil in 2 Tbsp. of carrier oil and massage into legs.

Health: Heals cuts and abrasions fast. Cypress is a safer alternative than antibiotics which leads to side effects including loss of probiotics.

Add 6 drops of cypress oil to warm bath water to relax after a long day. You may also like to add a couple of drops to your pillow to create a good night's sleep.

Dilute cypress oil with equal parts carrier oil such as coconut or jojoba oil to treat arthritis, cramps, asthma, bronchitis, cough or cold, carpal tunnel, and heavy periods. Massage oil mixture into effected area 2–3 times daily, depending on your needs.

Reduce phlegm by adding 6 drops of cypress oil to boiling water. Place a towel over your head and breathe in the steam for 5–15 minutes.

Household: Ideal for deodorizing rooms. Add a few drops to your diffuser for a great boost of fresh air.

> *Add 7 drops cypress, 5 drops eucalyptus, 4 drops lemon, and 6 drops of pine to a 1 oz spray bottle of water for a disinfecting and uplifting room spray.*

Add 5–10 drops of cypress oil to water and spray the mixture on curtains, sheets, and couches. Ideal for spraying on shoes, hats, and jackets to eliminate bacterial growth and body odor.

Add 5 to 10 drops of cypress oil to your laundry detergent to leave clothes bacteria-free and smelling fresh. Add it to a spray bottle for spraying on kitchen and bathroom surfaces.

DILL

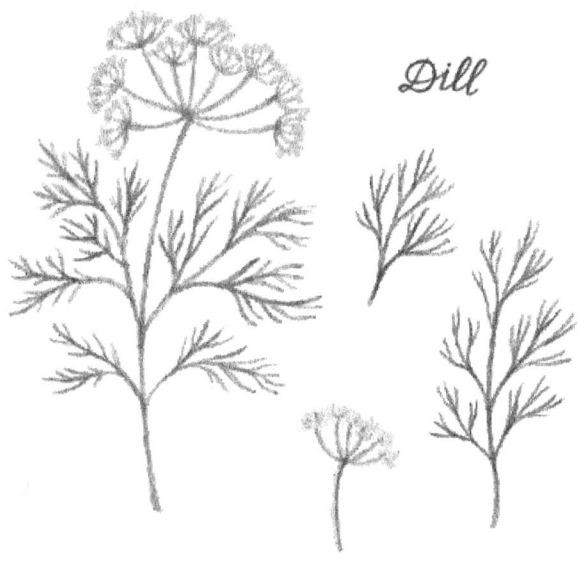

Dill

> *Herby, fresh, tangy. calming, and improves digestion.*

Anti-spasmodic, carminative, digestive, disinfectant, and sedative. Relieves spasms, eliminate excess gas, promotes healthy digestion, prohibits infections, increases secretion of milk, soothes hypersensitivity and anxiety. Increases perspiration.

Blends well with: Bergamot, lemon, lime, orange, marjoram, caraway, nutmeg, and oregano.

> *"The doctor of the future will give no medicine, but will interest his patients in the care of the human frame, in diet, and in the cause and prevention of disease." -Thomas Edison, Inventor*

Diffuse: Dill is useful for eliminating anxiety, tension, anger, and depression. It also aids a good night's sleep. Place 3 - 4 drops of oil in your diffuser.

Health: Dill can be used in a diluted form and applied to the scalp to protect hair and scalp from infections and lice. Add a few drops to your shampoo and conditioner.

Add your own recipes and tips here:

> *"The next major advance in the health of the American people will be determined by what the individual is willing to do for himself." - John Knowles, Former President of the Rockefeller Foundation*

EUCALYPTUS

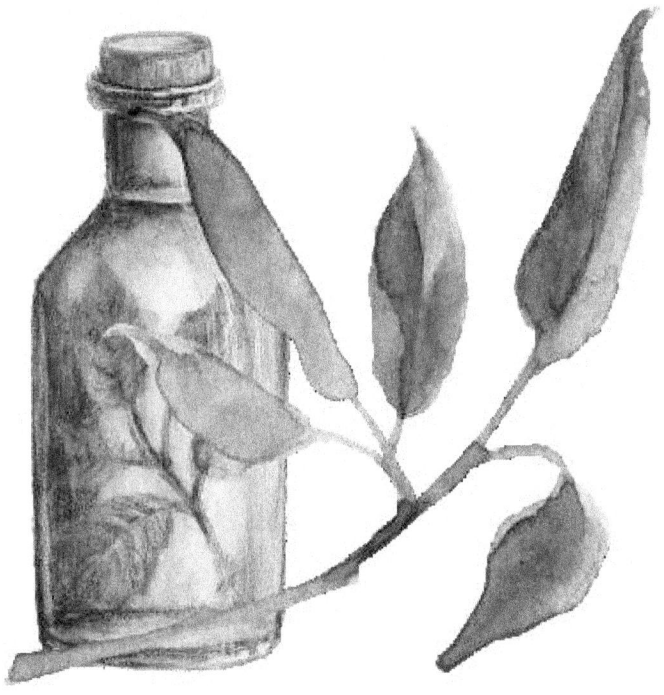

> **The healing witch:** *Helpful in recuperation after illnesses. Apply daily to the throat, forehead, wrists and bathwater. Ideal for purifications spells.*

Eucalyptus essential oil is used in classrooms to increase student performance. With rejuvenating and detoxifying qualities, eucalyptus oil is a popular addition to rubs, rash creams, and cosmetics.

A small town in Australia discovered that eucalyptus oil could be converted into a gas to light homes, and that they had stumbled upon one of the most powerful forms of natural medicine.

Cleansing, respiratory problems, and skin. Anti-inflammatory, antispasmodic, decongestant, deodorant, antiseptic, and antibacterial. Treatment of wounds, muscle pain, dental care, skin care, diabetes, fever, and intestinal germs.

Blends well with: Cannabis, cardamom, ginger, helichrysum, peppermint, rosemary, lemon, lavender, jasmine, lemon oil, cedarwood, thyme, frankincense oil, chamomile, geranium, grapefruit, juniper, lime, marjoram, orange, and tea tree oil.

Diffuse: Eucalyptus oil alleviates exhaustion and fatigue. Rejuvenates the spirits of those feeling sick. The refreshing scent can inspire alertness and alleviates stress. Add 3-4 drops to a diffuser and breathe in the clean, calming scent.

Massage: Add 2-3 drops into a carrier oil like castor oil then massage onto the chest. Eucalyptus oil's anti-inflammatory relieves symptoms of congestion.

For further results, massage mixture onto the skin after a shower.

Beauty: Add a drop or two to a facial cleanser or body lotion to rejuvenate the skin.

Add a few drops of eucalyptus oil with some coconut oil to give your hair a moisturizing treatement. A great treat for dandruff and an itchy scalp. Eucalyptus is also used as a natural remedy for a healthier alternative to lice treatments.

Health: Eucalyptus essential oil has antibacterial and antiseptic qualities, and when massaged onto the chest and used as a vapor rub or inhalant, it is beneficial in clearing the lungs and reducing inflammation. It is best applied to both the chest and the back.

For colds and flu, pour boiling water into a bowl and add 10 drops of eucalyptus oil. Placing a towel over your head, inhale for 5 – 15 minutes.

Combine a few drops of eucalyptus oil, peppermint oil, and coconut oil for a homemade vapor rub.

Mix 1-2 drops with warm water then gargle to combat a sore throat.

The vasodilating and relaxing qualities also benefit diabetics.

To fight a fever, combine a few drops with peppermint oil with water and spray on the body for a deodorant and a temperature reducer.

Household: Eucalyptus essential oil kills bacteria and germs in the air, keeping the environment of the rooms clean and sterilized. Also used to cleanse surfaces to kill bacteria.

Use as an air freshener to destroy airborne bacteria.

Add a few drops of eucalyptus oil to laundry detergent, mop water, toilet cleaner, window cleaner.

Make a spray by adding a few drops of eucalyptus oil to water and spray pet's bedding.

Mix eucalyptus oil with lemon oil or tea tree oil for an anti-stink spray. Ideal for spraying bins and toilets.

Add a few drops to your vacuum cleaner and clothes dryer filters to freshen and sanitize. Eucalyptus oil is also great for killing mold in your home. Mix eucalyptus with other oils like clove and tea tree oil to cleanse air-conditioners and maintain a mold-free environment.

Notes:

Eucalyptus oil is highly effective in removing spots on your carpet, sofa, clothes, curtains, including most other fabrics. Do a spot test to make sure the oil doesn't react strangely with the material you treat. Ideal for removing gum off shoes or fabric.

FENNEL

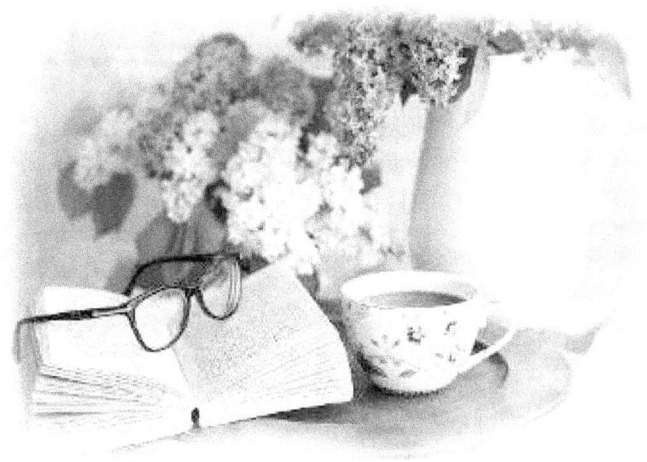

Fennel essential oil fights free radical damage and kills strains of bacteria and pathogenic fungi. Warm, sweet, licorice-like, and earthy.

Circulation, metabolism, improves digestion. Antiseptic, anti-spasmodic, carminative, depurative, diuretic, expectorant, laxative, and stimulant. Protects wounds, soothes spasms, increases appetite, removes excess gas, purifies the blood, increases urination, and promotes a regulated menstrual cycle. Defends against cough and cold, increases milk secretion, helps with constipation, and is good for stomach and spleen health.

Blends well with: Rose, orange, geranium, ylang-ylang, lavender essential oil, grapefruit, sandalwood essential oil, cypress, and sage.

Diffuse: Fennel can be added to many different diffuser formulas to boost aromatic and therapeutic benefits.

Diffuse to create a cozy, aromatic effect. A wonderful oil to diffuse when blended with rose and orange.

For relaxation, combine 3 drops of fennel essential oil with 4 drops of lavender oil in your diffuser.

Massage: Rub fennel essential oil on your stomach or the bottom of your feet to for digestive relief. Using a carrier oil helps prevent it from evaporating too quickly.

Calming massage. Blend 4 drops fennel essential oil, 4 drops clary sage essential oil, 2 drops geranium essential oil, and 1 drop melissa essential oil in 15 mL of coconut oil or almond oil.

Beauty: As it is both astringent and cleansing, it is helpful in addressing mature skin and in balancing dry or oily skin types.

Health: To calm an upset belly, blend 4 drops of fennel oil, 3 drops peppermint oil, 2 drops ginger essential oil, and 1 drop nutmeg essential oil in 15 mL of castor oil. Massage over abdomen.

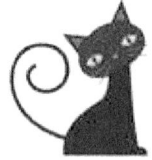 **Add your own recipes and notes here:**

FRANKINCENSE

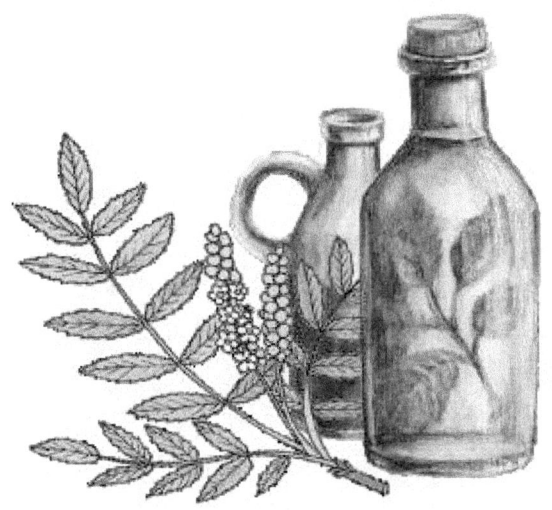

> **The sacred witch:** *One of the most sacred essential oils. Used to anoint magical tools and the altar. A strong purifier used in purification rituals, and blessings.*

Frankincense has always been synonymous with spirituality. The clean, citrus-terpenic fragrance of frankincense oil is entwined in ancient myth and sacred rituals. Frankincense oil uses include stress-relieving bath soak; natural household cleaner; natural hygiene product; anti-aging and wrinkle fighter; relieving the symptoms of indigestion; scar, stretch mark or acne remedy. It's a natural cold or flu medicine and can relieve inflammation and pain.

Clean, resinous, woody, balsamic. Frankincense oil is used by either inhaling the oil or absorbing it through the skin, usually mixed with a carrier oil, such as jojoba oil. Be careful not to apply it to broken skin. Emotional support, skin health. Antiseptic, disinfectant, astringent, cicatrisant, cytophylactic, emenagogue, expectorant, sedative, tonic, uterine, digestive, ans a diuretic. Protects wounds from becoming septic, fights infections, induces contractions in gums, muscles, and blood vessels, and removes excess gas, heals scars, keeps cells healthy and promotes regeneration. Promotes digestion, increases urination, regulates menstrual cycles, cures coughs, and colds, soothes anxiety and inflammation, and ensures good health of the uterus.

Blends well with: Grapefruit oil, bergamot oil, basil oil, black pepper oil, neroli oil, sandalwood oil, cedarwood, orange, lemon, bergamot, lavender, myrrh, cypress, rose, ylang ylang, clary sage, and geranium oil.

Diffuse: When inhaled, frankincense reduces heart rate and high blood pressure. It has anti-anxiety and depression-reducing abilities, but unlike prescription medications, it does not have negative side effects.

Diffusing 4 drops of frankincense essential oil and 3 drops of lavender lowers levels of anxiety and stress that can keep you up at night. It has a calming, grounding scent that can naturally help you to fall asleep.

Meditation Blend: Diffuse 8 drops frankincense oil, 6 drops sandalwood oil, and 4 drops cedarwood.

Massage: Add 5 drops of frankincense oil to any massage oil to soothe the skin, and relax the entire body and mind.

Meditation Blend 2: 4 drops frankincense oil, 4 drops sandalwood oil, 4 drops cedarwood oil in 30 mL of jojoba oil for a relaxing massage.

Beauty: Frankincense oil promotes regeneration of healthy cells and also keeps the existing cells and tissues healthy.

Add a drop to your skincare cream to help add luster to your skin. Frankincense also has the ability to strengthen skin and improve tone, elasticity, defense mechanisms against bacteria or blemishes, and appearance as someone ages. It helps tone and lift skin, reduces the appearance of scars and acne, and heals wounds.

Mix 5 drops of frankincense to one tablespoon of unscented oil such as coconut oil then apply directly to the skin. Be sure to do a patch area test first to test for possible allergic reactions.

> *Health: Make your own toothpaste by mixing a few drops of frankincense oil with coconut oil and baking soda.*

Use frankincense essential oil to provide relief from coughing. It can also help eliminate phlegm in the lungs. It also acts as an anti-inflammatory in the nasal passages, making breathing easier, even for those with allergies or asthma. Add 6 drops to a cloth and inhale for the respiratory benefits or use a diffuser.

Household: Frankincense is an antiseptic and disinfectant, eliminating cold and flu germs from the home and the body naturally. It can be used in place of chemical household cleaners. Add 6 drops of frankincense, 4 drops of orange, and 4 drops of lemon to water in a spray bottle. Shake before using.

Use in a diffuser to help reduce indoor pollution and deodorize and disinfect your home.

GERANIUM

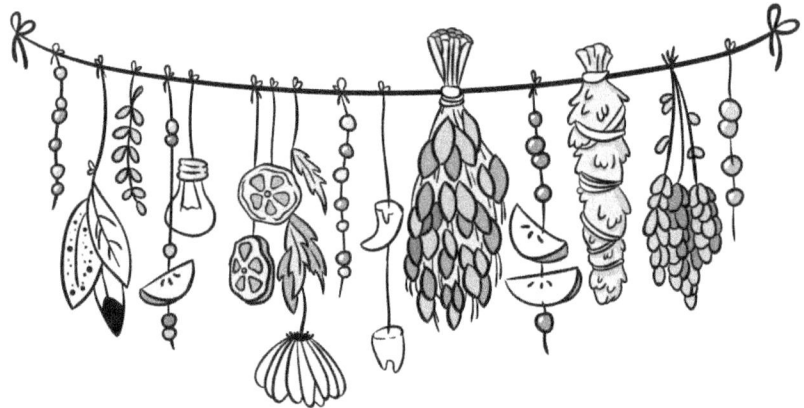

> *This sweet-smelling oil can also uplift your mood, lessen fatigue and promote emotional wellness. Herbaceous, green, floral, sweet, dry. Insect repellent, calming, improved skin and hair health.*

Astringent, tonic, cicatrisant, cytophylactic, diuretic, deodorant, haemostatic, styptic, vermifuge, and vulnerary. Induce tightening of the gums, muscles, skin and blood vessels and in stopping hemorrhage, scar healing, promotion of cell growth, and increased urination. Stops body odor, tone up the body.

Blends well with: Angelica, bergamot, basil, cedarwood, lavender, neroli, lime, orange, lemon, jasmine, grapefruit, chamomile, vetiver, peppermint, sandalwood, and rosemary Oil.

How to use.

Diffuse: The sweet and floral smell of geranium oil calms and relaxes the body and mind. Why not put your feet up and read a book. A cup of Jasmine tea might also be nice.

Add three to four drops to your diffuser to help relieve pent-up stress and tension.

Add 2 drops of jasmine, 2 drops of chamomile, and 2 drops of clary sage to create an uplifting floral bouquet. Add peppermint for a minty, effervescent kick for a quick boost anytime of the day.

Massage: It's best to dilute geranium oil with a carrier oil when you are applying it directly to the skin. Mix geranium oil with equal parts coconut, jojoba or olive oil.

For a sensual massage, try blending geranium with either sandalwood or vetiver with your favorite carrier oil.

Beauty: Rather than paying all that money to rub toxic chemicals over your body, applying a small amount of geranium oil to help you achieve flawless skin. The oil helps in the treatment of acne, dermatitis and skin diseases. Being a powerful cicatrizant, it helps the scars and other spots on the skin fade. It facilitates blood circulation just below the surface of the skin and helps promote a uniform distribution of melanin.

Blend a teaspoon of coconut oil with 4 - 5 drops of geranium oil, then rub the mixture onto your skin.

You can also add 2 drops of geranium oil to your daily face or body wash.

Add 5 drops of geranium oil to a spray bottle and mix it with ½ a cup of water to create a natural and beneficial perfume.

Add a couple of drops into your shampoo or conditioner to bring out your hair's natural shine.

Health: Geranium oil can prevent nose and throat infections, as it contains several chemicals that have antibiotic-like effects.

Diffuse or massage into the throat and neck area. Add a little under your nose.

Geranium oil has the power to fight nerve pain when it's applied to the skin. To fight nerve pain with geranium oil, create a massage oil with 3 drops of geranium oil in a tablespoon of coconut oil. Massage into your skin, focusing on the areas where you feel pain or tension.

Geranium oil has shown to be a safer and more effective ingredient for anti-inflammatory medication.

Household: Geranium oil is used as a natural bug repellant.

To make your own bug repellant, mix 10 drops of geranium oil with ½ cup of water and spray it on your body – a much safer option than store bought sprays that are filled with toxic chemicals. Add baking soda to this mixture and apply to insect bites to stop itching.

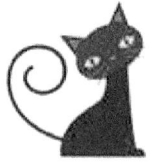 Add your own recipe here:

GINGER

The passionate witch: *A tropical aphrodisiac. Induces passion.*

Ginger essential oil is often used to treat nausea, upset stomachs, menstrual disorders, inflammation and respiratory conditions. When used in aromatherapy, it is also known for bringing on feelings of courageousness and self-assurance, which is why it's known as "the oil of empowerment." Spicy, hot and distinctive.

Grounding, antioxidant, digestive support. Analgesic, carminative, antiemetic, antiseptic, antispasmodic, bactericidal, cephalic, expectorant, febrifuge, rubefacient, stimulant, stomachic, laxative, sudorific, and a tonic. Eases vomiting, protect from wounds becoming septic, and relax spasm. Inhibits bacterial growth, eliminate gas, and improve brain and memory function. Expel phlegm & catarrh. Break fevers, clear bowels, bring color to the skin, improve stomach health, and promote sweating, removes toxins from the body.

Blends well with: Neroli, orange, geranium, coriander, clove, cedarwood, sandalwood, rose, mandarin, lime, lemon and others of the kind.

Diffuse: When used as aromatherapy, ginger essential oil is able to relieve feelings of anxiety, anxiousness, depression and exhaustion.

> *Diffuse a drop or 2 while you are driving on a long trip to keep your focus on the road. Also helps settle motion sickness.*

Diffuse 2 to 3 drops in your home or in your office to elevate your spirits and get you through the lethargic hours of the afternoon when you feel tired.

For nausea, diffuse 3 drops of ginger oil.

For easy and comfortable breathing, use 4 drops of ginger with a few drops of cardamom essential oil plus 2 drops of thyme essential oil.

Massage: A little goes a long way. When massaged into skin, use diluted with a carrier oil.

For muscle and joint pain, massage 1 to 3 drops of the oil on the needed area twice daily.

For nausea, apply 1 to 2 drops over the stomach.

> *Soft Tissue Massage: 4 drops ginger, 6 drops peppermint, 6 drops Eucalyptus, and 2 drops frankincense in 30 mL of carrier oil.*

Ginger essential oil has long been used for increasing libido in both men and women.

Health: To improve blood circulation and heart health, rub 1 to 2 drops of ginger essential oil over the heart twice daily.

To aid digestion and get rid of toxins, add 2 to 3 drops of ginger oil to warm bath water and take a long soak.

Apply a drop of ginger oil to a tissue or cotton ball for enhancing balance and as a quick support for discomfort.

> *Mix 1 drop ginger oil with 3 drops of chamomile and add to a warm bath to soothe an upset belly.*

How To Make Ginger Essential Oil.

Step 1 – Rinse 1 cup of chopped fresh ginger and let it dry for up to 1-2 hours.

Step 2 – Add 2 cups of olive oil to an oven-safe bowl, then grate the dry ginger into the oil and mix.

Step 3 – Place the bowl in the oven for 2 hours on a low heat (170 degrees Fahrenheit).

Step 4 – Strain the ginger and oil mixture through the cheesecloth and into a glass jar.

Step 5 – Store in an airtight glass jar away from sunlight or heat for up to six months.

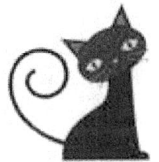 **Add your own recipe or tips here:**

GRAPEFRUIT

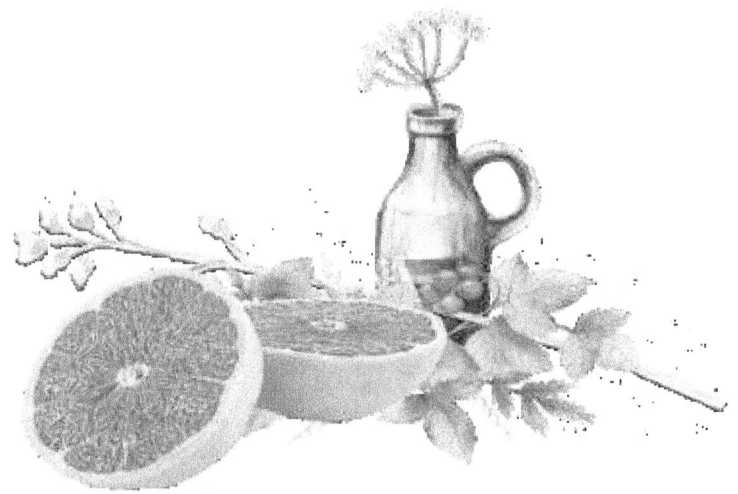

Grapefruit oil is extracted from the peel which holds a range of beneficial compounds. As one of the most versatile essential oils, the aroma of grapefruit oil is clean, fresh and a little bit bitter.

Stimulating, alertness, cleansing, skin health, appetite suppressant. Diuretic, disinfectant, stimulant, antidepressant, antiseptic, aperitif, lymphatic, and a tonic. Stimulate urination, fight infections, reduce depression, uplift mood. Protects wounds from becoming septic. Increasing the elimination of toxins.

> ***Blends well with:*** *Basil oil, orange oil, peppermint oil, bergamot oil, eucalyptus oil, tea tree oil, patchouli, and lemon.*

Diffuse: Stress Buster. The smell of grapefruits is uplifting, soothing and clarifying. Grapefruit essential oil can increase your mental focus, giving you a natural pick-me-up. When inhaled, its stimulating effects also make it effective for reducing headaches, sleepiness, "brain fog," mental fatigue and even your mood.

It's known to bust stress and works great when it's diffused, added to bath water. You can also dab on the skin like perfume. Add several drops of the oil to a clean cotton ball with a touch of coconut oil, then apply to your wrists, neck or chest.

Hungover? To help alleviate the symptoms of withdrawal, diffuse 2 - 3 drops of grapefruit essential oil in your home.

To eliminate unpleasant odors in the kitchen and bathroom, diffuse grapefruit oil along with other citrus scents like lemon oil and orange oil. While your house fills with a clean scent, you also eliminate odor-causing bacteria from the air.

Grapefruit also works as a mild, natural antidepressant while it calms the nerves.

Massage: Should be diluted with a carrier oil like coconut or jojoba oil in a 1:1 ratio before applying to skin. Combine the 2, and then rub them onto any area in need, including sore muscles, acne-prone skin or your abdomen to improve digestion.

Beauty: *As a natural acne treatment or skin salve. Add 3 drops of grapefruit oil to a teaspoon of coconut or jojoba oil and apply to the skin.*

Health: Grapefruit's active ingredients are beneficial to boost metabolism and reduce your appetite. When mixed with patchouli oil, grapefruit oil is known to lower cravings and hunger, which makes it a great to lose weight fast in a healthy way.

Grapefruit oil is known for lowering sugar cravings while helping you kick sugar addiction when inhaled. Sniff the oil directly from the bottle when needed.

A natural remedy for PMS cramps, headaches, bloating, fatigue and muscle aches and pains. Add a few drops to your bath. Place some on your shirt collar. **Digestion.** Make a homemade massage lotion with 4 drops of grapefruit added coconut or jojoba oil and rub the mixture onto your abdomen.

> ***Household:*** *Use a small amount of grapefruit essential oil on wooden surfaces, countertops, floors, in household appliances, and bins to kill bacteria and odor naturally.*

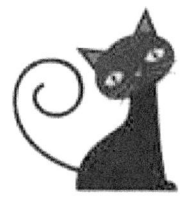 Add your own recipes and tips here:

> *"The art of healing comes from nature and not from the physician. Therefore, the physician must start from nature with an open mind." -Paracelsus*

HELICHRYSUM

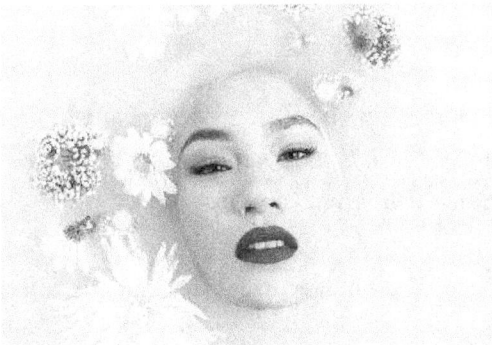

The go-to oil for skin beautifying and restorative serums, helichrysum is potent, safe, and exceptionally effective. Helichrysum oil is described as a sweet and fruity smell, with honey or nectar overtones. In clinical studies, the flavonoids and phloroglucinols of helichrysum oil showed inhibition of harmful bacteria, fungi and viruses, even powerful enough to help decrease the risk of contracting the HIV.

Improves metabolism, healthy skin. Fights allergies, dissolves and clears blood clots, reduces inflammation from fever. Nervous system health. Reduces inflammation, clears phlegm and reduces coughs, heals scars, protects wounds from becoming septic, stimulates proper bile discharge, kills fungus. Stimulating urination and regeneration of new cells.

Blends well with: Bergamot, black pepper, chamomile, citrus oils, clary sage, clove, cypress, geranium, juniper, lavender, neroli, oakmoss, oregano, rose, rosemary, tea tree, thyme, vetiver, and ylang ylang.

Diffuse: When diffused, the oil exudes a very calming aroma. This plays an essential role on your emotional state, and helps shake off mental fatigue.

Diffuse 4 – 5 drops of helichrysum to aid soothing nerves and calming the heart.

Massage: To use helichrysum essential oil for soothing and healing the skin, combine with a carrier oil like coconut or jojoba oil and rub the mixture onto the face.

> *Prevents hives, blemishes, rashes, and shaving irritation. Applying helichrysum mixed with lavender oil can help cool and soothe any itching associated with hives.*

Apply 2-4 drops of undiluted oil directly on the skin to the affected area or desired location.

Or – 2 – 4 drops on sore bodies to soothe, just add it to your favorite massage oil and rub.

Beauty: The go-to oil for skin beautifying and restorative serums, this extraordinary distillation has a rich, herbaceous, honey-like bouquet.

To battle acne pimples, wrinkles as well as skin blemishes, apply 1 – 2 drops of the oil to the designated area. Using carrier oil is advised.

> ***Skin Rejuvenation blend:*** *12 drops helichrysum essential oil, 6 drops carrot seed essential oil, 6 drops rosemary oil in 15 ml rosehip oil, and 1 teaspoon of coconut oil.*

Health: Being an antitussive, helichrysum oil gives relief from coughs that are stimulated by phlegm in the respiratory tracts or by itchiness in the throat caused by infections.

JASMINE

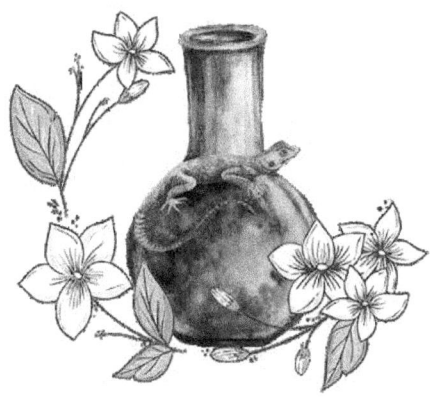

> **The mysterious witch:** *Symbol of the Moon, mysteries of the night.*
> *Jasmine oil is used in spells to attract love. The scent also helps*
> *you to relax, sleep, and facilitates in childbirth. It is sometimes used*
> *for meditation and general anointing purposes.*

Jasmine oil is one of the most popular scents used in perfumery. Balances the mood, healthy skin. Fights depression and uplifts mood, protects wounds, cures sexual dysfunctions. Increases libido. Reduces spasms, heals scars, relief from phlegm and coughs, increases breast milk, regulates menstrual cycles. Eases labor pains. Sedating inflammation and nervous disturbances.

Blends well with: Bergamot, sandalwood, rose, orange, lemon, limes, grapefruit, and ylang ylang.

Diffuse: Jasmine essential oil calms down the body, mind, and soul while bringing forth positive and constructive emotions. It gives relief from anxiety, stress, annoyance, anger, and depression Known to increase sensuality.

Inhaling jasmine oil, either directly or by diffusing it in your home, helps clear mucus and bacteria within the nasal passages. To diffuse jasmine oil at home, combine 3 drops each of - lavender oil or frankincense oil.

Massage: It doesn't need to be combined with a carrier oil and instead is recommended to be used undiluted for the best results.

Beauty: Instead of using expensive store-bought perfumes, dab jasmine oil onto your wrists and neck as a natural, chemical-free alternative. Jasmine oil has a flowery smell, and a little will go a long way, so only use only 1 - 2 drops. Mix with a carrier oil for best results.

Health: Jasmine oil contains active ingredients, such as benzaldehyde, benzoic acid, and benzyl benzoate which fight harmful bacteria and viruses in the body and on the skin, helping prevent sickness, irritation, fungus and viral infections.

Jasmine oil aids in balancing hormones naturally and has been used successfully used to increase production of breast milk. Applying jasmine oil to the skin helps to prevent stretch marks and scarring.

To create a natural vapor rub, mix jasmine with a carrier oil and eucalyptus oil. Massage it onto your chest, temples, neck, and anywhere else you experience pain.

Try adding Jasmine oil to your bath water. Rub it onto your skin during your morning shower to help you ease into the day.

It is also used to free people from narcotic and other addictions.

JUNIPER BERRY

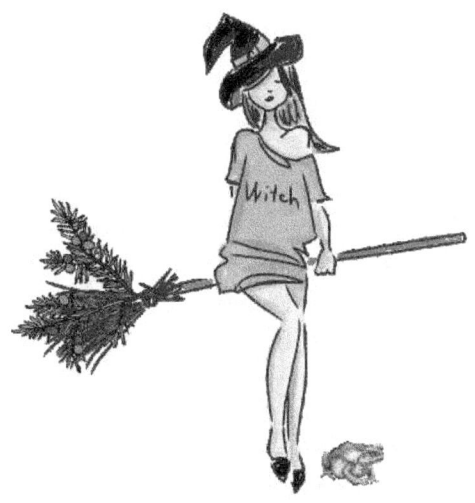

> *During the Medieval period, juniper berries were believed to help ward off evil witches.*

Juniper berries were seen as protectors of health — both emotional and physical health. Fresh yet warm, terpenic, bittersweet, woody, conifer.

Stress relief, cleansing, skin toner, kidney/urinary support. Antiseptic, sudorific, antirheumatic, antispasmodic, stimulating, astringent, carminative, and a diuretic. Protects wounds from becoming septic, increases sweating, cures rheumatism and arthritis, purifies blood, eliminates spasms, stimulates functions, and is good for the stomach. Stronger gums and stops hemorrhaging, reduces excess gas, promotes urination, brings color to the skin, promotes quick healing of wounds.

Blends will with: Bergamot essential oil, grapefruit essential oil, lime essential oil; cedarwood essential oil, cypress essential oil, pine, geranium essential oil, clary sage essential oil, and vetiver.

Diffuse: Juniper essential oil works to support clear breathing, detoxification, and cleansing. When diffused indoors, it absorbs odors from your home while also purifying the air your family breathes.

Use juniper berry oil at home, diffusing it throughout your bedroom. Dab some on your wrists diluted with a carrier oil. Sprinkle it on your clothes for an uplifting perfume. Add a few drops directly to your bath water for a calming, healing soak.

The smell of juniper berries reduces physical and emotional stress. 4 drops is usually ample to enhance the overall ambiance of your home or office.

Massage: You should always dilute juniper oil with a carrier oil like coconut oil (1:1 ratio) before applying it to your skin.

Mix several drops of Juniper essential oil with 1 to 2 teaspoons of coconut or jojoba oil. Massage the mixture into affected areas for relief.

Balance Blend: 5 drops juniper berry, 4 drops rosemary oil, 4 drops geranium oil, 4 drops cypress oil, and 2 drops of lavender essential oil in a tablespoon of jojoba oil.

Joint Blend: 8 drops juniper oil, 4 drops Eucalyptus oil, 4 drops rosemary oil, 4 drops marjoram oil, and 2 drops ginger oil in a tablespoon of coconut oil or castor oil.

Beauty: Use 1 - 2 drops mixed with a carrier oil as a gentle astringent or moisturizer after washing your face.

For skin health, mix one drop in your facial moisturizer.

Health: Add juniper berry to your bathwater to help treat blemishes and foot odors and fungus.

To support a healthy system, add 4 - 5 drops to warm bath water and take a relaxing soak.

> **Household:** *Consider adding several drops of juniper berry to your laundry detergent mix so the smell lingers on your clothes and linens.*

Run several drops through your washing machine or dishwasher and replace commercial cleaning products — which usually contain multiple harsh chemicals — with natural antibacterial juniper oil mixed with water.

To help prevent and reduce bacterial strains from spreading throughout your home, use juniper berry on kitchen and bathroom surfaces.

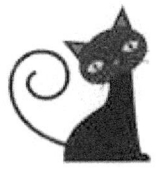 **Add your own recipes and tips here:**

LAVENDER

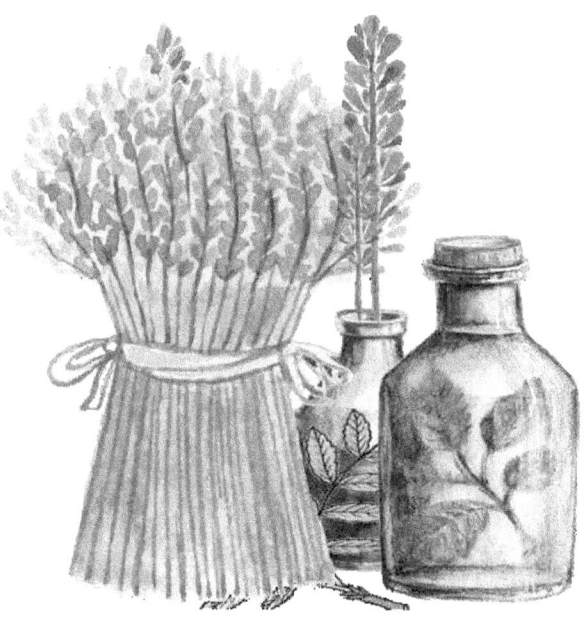

The sexy witch: *Used to arouse sexual desire in men, and purifying spells and rituals.*

According to the ancient healing system of Ayurveda, by balancing "wind," lavender oil will assist in slowing down the overly active mind and will support tranquility and peacefulness.

By balancing "fire," lavender oil will decrease excess heat in the body and mind and will support clarity and brightness of presence. By balancing "phlegm," lavender oil helps to lighten tendencies toward sluggishness, complacency, and melancholy.

Ayurvedic medicine is one of the world's oldest holistic healing systems. It was developed more than 3,000 years ago in India. It is based on the belief that health and wellness depend on a healthy balance between the mind, body, and spirit.)

Lavender is mood-uplifting and supports heightened energy. Lavender essential oil gives luster to the skin, balance to the body and happiness to the mind. Lavender oil has also been used in the making of perfumes. Light, floral and powdery. Universal oil, calming, stress relief, skin health, headache relief. Sleep-inducing, analgesic, disinfectant, anti-inflammatory, antiseptic, and antifungal. Pain relief, urine flow, respiratory disorders, skin care, hair care, blood circulation, indigestion, and immune system health.

Blends well with: Bergamot, Chamomile, Clary sage, Geranium, Jasmine, Lemon, Mandarin, Orange, Patchouli, Pine, Tangerine, Thyme, Rosemary, Rosewood, Nutmeg, and Ylang Ylang.

Diffuse: Diffuse lavender your home to help you relax and to refresh the whole family. When you have guests over, their first comments are likely to be compliments on the fragrance of your home.

Do you suffer from anxious moods? For the best results, you need to diffuse at least 4 drops.

To relieve stress and improve sleep, place a diffuser by your bed and diffuse the oils while you sleep or in the family room while you're reading or winding down in the evening.

> *Diffusing lavender or inhaling it directly from the bottle can also help to relieve headaches.*

To relieve stress, anxiety, and improve sleep, diffuse lavender or inhale it directly from the bottle.

If you have kids, lavender oil is ideal. Use it in your diffuser while the kids are playing, or place a drop in their hands for direct palm inhalation before leaving for school.

Rest: 4 drops lavender, 2 drops chamomile and 1 drop cedarwood. Add to a massage oil or to your diffuser.

Massage: Blend 4 drops mandarin, 2 drops grapefruit, 2 drops lavender and 2 drops Roman chamomile. Add to 1 Tbsp. of coconut oil and massage into skin.

Beauty: If you are having issues with greasy and oily hair, adding lavender to your shampoo will help. At the same time, it can prevent dandruff formation.

Skin Repair Blend: 4 drops lavender, 4 drops helichrysum, and 2 drops rose in 1 Tbsp. of aloe vera gel.

You can also add lavender oil to your face or body wash. Mix lavender oil with frankincense essential oil and applying it to your skin in the morning after you shower, then again before bed. This will help reduce inflammation and signs of aging and dark spots.

To use lavender for skin health, combine 3–4 drops with ½ teaspoon of coconut or jojoba oil and massage the mixture into the area of concern.

Homemade perfume. Add 2 drops of lavender oil to a spray bottle with about ½ cup of water. Shake up the spray bottle and then spray away.

Health: If you are suffering from increased levels of anxiety, mix with water in a spray bottle. Use this at your home, car, and office, and it may help you reduce the feelings of nervousness.

For burn relief and to heal cuts, scrapes or wounds, mix 4–5 drops of lavender with ½ teaspoon of coconut oil and apply the mixture to the area of concern. You can use your fingers or a clean cotton ball.

One of the most effective natural headache remedies is combing 2 drops each of lavender oil with peppermint oil with a couple of drops of carrier oil and rubbing the mixture into the back of your neck and the temples.

If you are feeling nauseous, or know that you are going to be traveling in a car of plane and are prone to motion sickness, spray some lavender oil on your skin and clothes, or rub it into your temples, neck, and palms.

Household: The smell of lavender essential oil is deadly to many types of bugs like mosquitoes, midges, and moths. Apply some lavender oil on the exposed skin or diffuse when outside.

Apply a drop or 2 to bedding, bottoms of the feet or to your pillows during bedtime in order to induce a feeling of calmness and to promote peaceful sleeping. You can also combine the oil with water in a simple spray bottom in order to freshen up the air in your office, home or car.

> *The same way you use lavender oil as a perfume; you can use it around your home as a natural, toxin-free air freshener.*

Spray lavender oil around your home or try diffusing it. To create a relaxing atmosphere in your bedroom before you fall asleep, try spraying the lavender oil and water mixture directly onto your bed sheets or pillow.

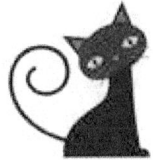

LEMON

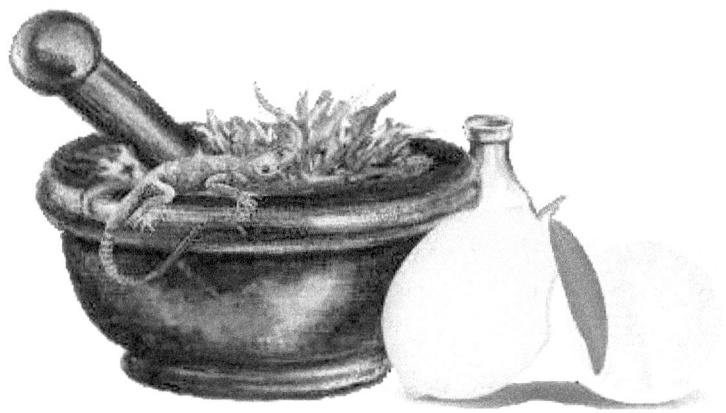

Lemon essential oil comes from cold-pressing the lemon peel, not the inner fruit. The peel is the most nutrient portion of the lemon regarding fat-soluble phytonutrients.

Ayurvedic medicine has been using both lemons and lemon essential oil to treat a wide spectrum of health conditions for well over 1,000 years.

Reminiscent of lemon blossom flowers freshly plucked from a lemon tree. Smells like pure citrusy-floral freshness! Energy, stimulating, respiratory support, improves digestion. Protects from wounds becoming septic, inhibiting viral and bacterial growth, strengthening gums, and stopping hair loss. Induces firmness in muscles, stops hemorrhage, fights infections, and cures fever.

> **Blends well with:** *Chamomile, eucalyptus, fennel, frankincense, geranium, juniper, lavender, neroli, rose, sandalwood, and ylang ylang*

Diffuse: If you are experiencing seasonal respiratory discomfort, diffusing in your home, office or vehicle may help you substantially. It may also help you with your overall respiratory function. Known for its bright, tangy, and pure scent, lemon essential oil can clear and refresh a fatigued mind quickly when added to your diffuser. When diffused, lemon has an uplifting and energizing effect. It may also improve your mood and encourage motivation.

Try a simple blend of lavender and lemon – 3 drops of each.

Mix 2 drops of each, lemon oil, lavender oil, neroli oil, and tea tree oil to freshen and purify the air.

Massage: Use a drop or 2 in your usual massage blend for an invigorating and uplifting massage.

Beauty: Added to your bath water, lemon delivers an aromatic, healing, stimulating and energizing bath.

Hair Rinse. Making a hair rinse is a quick rejuvenating treat for your hair. Mix 1/4 cup of lemon juice with a cup of warm water and pour it over your hair after shampooing. Rub it through your hair before rinsing out at the end of the shower.

Scalp Cream. Blend 1 Tbsp. of olive oil with 5 drops of lemon essential oil. Rub this mixture well into the scalp and leave it on for 1-2 hours, or even overnight. In the morning, rinse your scalp thoroughly.

> ***Castor Oil.*** *Mixing castor oil and lemon juice is a popular solution for dandruff and other inflammatory conditions that affect the scalp.*

Honey. Blend honey and lemon juice for a hair mask is an effective way to improve the strength of your hair, reduce oiliness, and boost luster.

Health: Promotes Fat-Loss – Putting 2 drops of lemon oil in your water 3x daily can support metabolism and weight loss.

> ***Only use food-grade 100% essential oils when consuming any essential oils.***

Immune Support – Lemon oil can support lymphatic drainage and help you overcome a cold fast, mix a few drops with coconut oil and rub it on your neck.

Lemon aromatherapy during pregnancy assistances in alleviating bouts of nausea and vomiting.

Household: Laundry – In case you leave your laundry sitting in the washer too long, just add a few drops of lemon to your wash to avoid that nasty, old-sock smell.

Clean greasy hands – If you have greasy hands from working on your car or bike, regular soap doesn't cut the mustard. Add a couple drops of lemon oil with your soap, that should do the trick.

> ***Wood and Silver Polish*** *– A lemon oil-soaked cloth will also help spruce up your tarnished silver and jewelry! Lemon oil is also an ideal wood cleaning.*

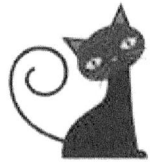 **Add your own recipe or tips here:**

LEMONGRASS

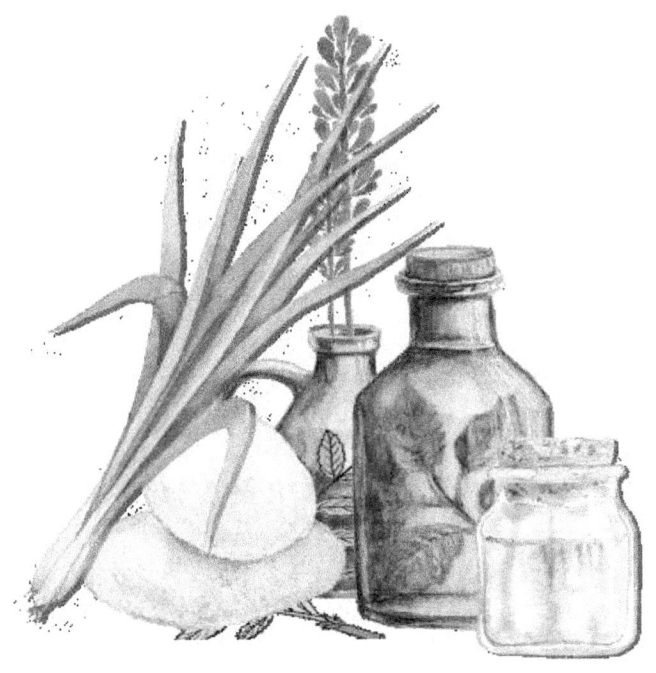

> **The spiritual witch:** *Lemongrass awakens psychic powers.*
> *Spiritualists and mediums use it to make contact with spirits in the*
> *in-between.*

As the name implies, lemongrass smells just like lemons, but it is milder, sweeter, and far less sour.

Lemongrass oil is often used in aromatherapy to relieve muscle pain, externally to kill bacteria, ward off insects, and reduce body aches and pains while assisting your digestive system.

Calming, improved digestion, complexion, insect repellent. Reduces pain, fights depression, reduces high fever, protects wounds from being septic, strengthens gums and hair and reduces hemorrhaging. Eliminates gas, reduces body odor, promotes urination, reduces fever, stops fungal infections, increases milk, soothes inflammation and cures nervous disturbances.

Blends well with: Basil, bergamot, black pepper, cedarwood, clary sage, coriander, cypress, fennel, geranium, ginger, grapefruit, lavender, lemon, marjoram, orange, patchouli, rosemary, tea tree, thyme, vetiver, and ylang ylang.

Diffuse: If you want to use lemongrass in your diffuser, you need no more than 4 drops in a regular diffuser.

Lemongrass oil boosts self-esteem, confidence, hope, mental strength, uplifts spirits, and fights depression.

By adding other oils like lavender and peppermint, you can customize your own natural fragrance.

Diffuse a blend of lemongrass oil, lavender oil, and cedar oil to promote emotional equilibrium.

Massage: Add two drops to your massage blend to balance the mind and emotions and energize the skin.

Beauty: Lemongrass oil can strengthen your hair follicles, so if you are struggling with hair loss or an itchy and irritated scalp, massage a few drops of lemongrass oil into your scalp for 2 minutes and then rinse. The soothing and bacteria-killing properties will leave your hair shiny and fresh.

> **Body scrub:** *Blend 10 drops of lemongrass oil with Epsom salt. Add enough coconut oil to saturate the salt. In the shower, rub the scrub over your body (including your face) then rinse.*

Health: For headache Relief. The soothing effects of lemongrass oil has the power to relieve the pain, pressure, or tension that can cause headaches. Try massaging diluted lemongrass oil on your temples and breathe in the relaxing lemony fragrance.

Foot soak: make your own foot soak by adding about 10 drops of lemongrass essential oil to warm water. This should relieve any muscle pain that you are feeling in your feet and it has antibacterial and antifungal effects too.

> **Household:** *For a super easy DIY insect repellent, add 40 drops of lemongrass essential oil to a spray bottle and the mosquitoes won't bother you.*

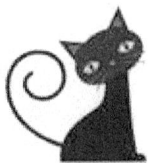 **Add your own recipes and tips here:**

LIME

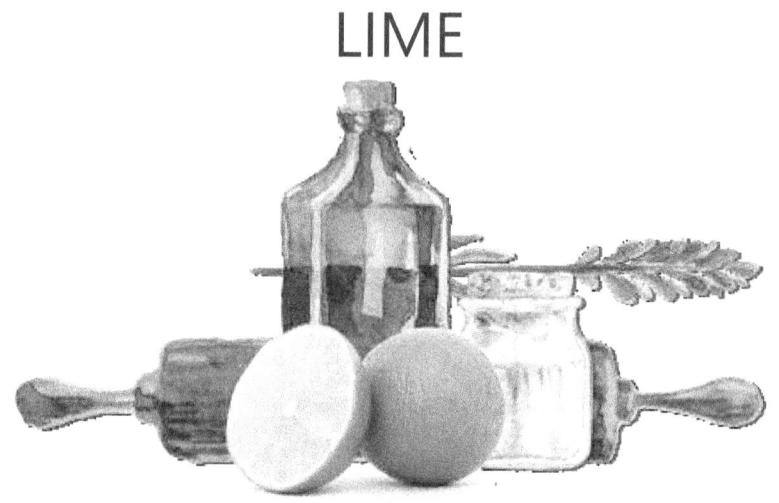

> *Lime's refreshing yet not-too-sweet properties can assist with enhancing mental clarity and alertness and can also promote feelings of positivity, calm and harmony.*

Antiviral, astringent, restorative, and a wellbeing tonic. Protect wounds from becoming septic, healing properties and boosts appetite. Kills bacteria, reduces a fever, stop hemorrhage, lifts general health.

Blends well with: Clary Sage, Lavender, Neroli, and Ylang-Ylang oil.

How to use.

Diffuse: Diffuse no more than 4 drops in order to induce an uplifting local environment. Use this at work in order to avoid feelings of lethargy in the afternoon.

> *Diffuse lime oil with grapefruit oil and lavender oil to soothe the nervous system, to boost mental clarity, and to help reduce stress and tension.*

Massage: Essence Blend: 8 drops lime oil, 8 drops frankincense oil, 2 drops patchouli oil and 2 drops of sandalwood oil in 1 tablespoon of jojoba oil or coconut oil.

Health: Lime essential oil tones up muscles, tissues, and skin as well as the various systems that function in the body, including the respiratory, circulatory, nervous, digestive, and excretory systems.

This tonic effect helps to retain youth for a long time and prevents the appearance of aging symptoms like hair loss, wrinkles, age spots, and muscle weakness.

2 drops lime in an aromatic bath can help soothe the digestive system and can help enhance muscle and joint health.

 **Add your own recipes and tips here:**

MANDARIN

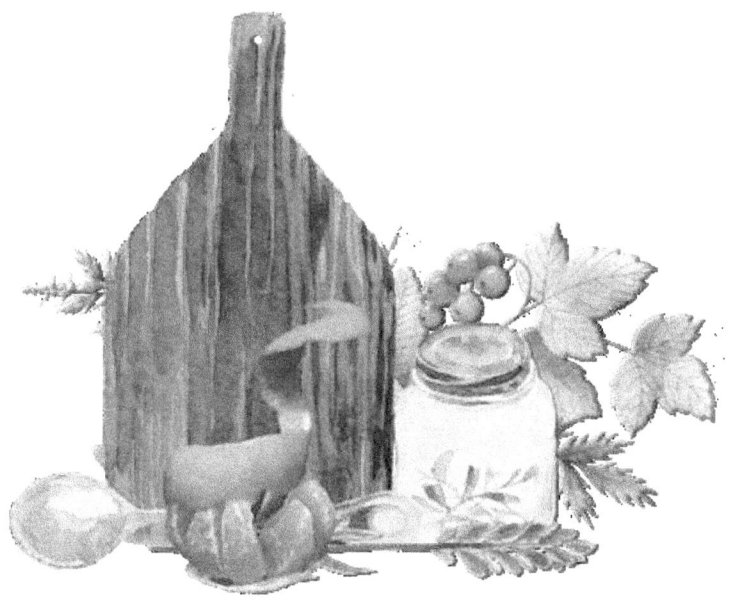

Dating back thousands of years to Chinese medicine, mandarin is known to be the most calming of all citrus essential oils.

Protects wounds from becoming septic, promotes growth, increases blood and lymph circulation, & regeneration of cells, purifies blood, facilitates digestion, and is good for the liver. Soothes inflammation and nervous afflictions. Toning the body.

Blends well with: Clary sage oil, vetiver oil, sandalwood oil, rose, geranium oil, jasmine oil, lavender oil, ylang-ylang oil, lime oil, grapefruit oil, bergamot oil, lemon oil; cinnamon oil, clove oil, and ginger.

Diffuse: Reach for mandarin any time you want to sweeten the bouquet of your diffuser blend.

Mandarin essential oil is ideal for soothing anxiety and nausea. Diffuse mandarin to shift a negative mood and promote contentment; the sweet and tangy bouquet is uplifting for all ages.

For variety, you can add some lavender, or other citrus oils like grapefruit, and bergamot for an uplifting mix. Add 10 drops mandarin oil, 2 drops rosemary, and 2 drops lavender for a calming blend.

Massage:

Belly Blend: 4 drops mandarin oil, 2 drops grapefruit oil, 2 drops lavender oil, and 2 drops chamomile oil in 1 tablespoon of coconut oil or another carrier oil.

Beauty: Add mandarin to your skin care formulations to smooth the skin and add natural beauty. Reduces the appearance of scars. Blend 1 drop lavender, 1 drop mandarin, and 1 drop neroli with a little almond oil. Apply to scars.

Health: It protects wounds from becoming septic as well as from other bacterial, fungal or viral infections. The essential oil of mandarin also promotes the growth of new cells and tissues, thereby helping to speed the healing time of wounds.

Household:

> *In the Laundry*: *Add several drops of mandarin oil to a clean damp washcloth and toss in the dryer to freshen linens.*

Air freshener: Add 10 drops mandarin oil and 2 drops rosemary and 2 drops lavender to a spray bottle for a rejuvenating and purifying air freshener.

MANUKA

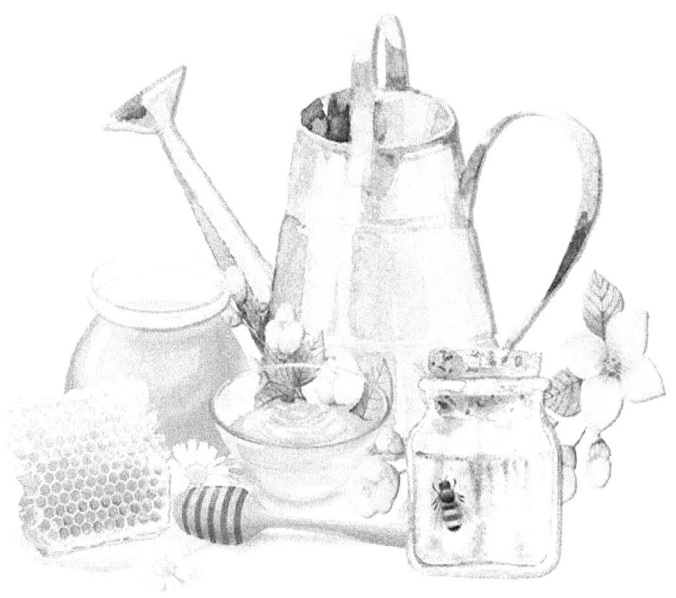

> *Manuka and its uses in aromatherapy were discovered only quite recently. However, its medicinal uses have been known for a long time among the original inhabitants of New Zealand, the country to which this tree is native.*

Antidandruff, an antidote to insect bites. Antibacterial and antiallergenic. Nervous relaxant. Treats dandruff, inhibit bacterial and fungal infections, sedate inflammation, check production of histamine and reduce allergic symptoms. Clears up scars and spots, promotes growth & regeneration of cells, reduces body odor.

Blends well with: Clove, Clary Sage, Geranium, Lavender, Marjoram, Nutmeg, Rosemary, and Ylang-Ylang.

Diffuse: Inhaling manuka essential oil can treat a variety of respiratory conditions including asthma, sinus congestion, and the symptoms of colds and the flu.

Manuka oil gives a relaxed feeling by fighting depression, anxiety, anger, stress, nervous afflictions, and disturbances.

Allergies: Diffuse manuka around your home for allergy relief.

Massage:

If you suffer with athlete's foot, apply manuka essential oil a couple of times a day for an effective natural remedy. Massage the oil into the feet morning and night then cover your feet with socks to ensure that the oil is well absorbed.

Treat joint and muscle pain by diluting manuka oil with a suitable carrier oil and making a soothing massage oil.

Health: Manuka essential oil can eliminate a variety of fungi and bacteria that thrive on the feet and toes and cause athlete's foot.

Foot soak: To fight fungi and bacteria, add 6 drops of manuka oil to a warm bowl of water and soak your feet for around 20 minutes every day.

Alternatively, add 8 – 10 drops of manuka essential oil to your bathwater several times a week or when needed.

Bites and stings: Dab a little manuka oil onto the affected area as soon as possible and you should feel instant relief, including a reduction in swelling, itching, and redness.

MARJORAM

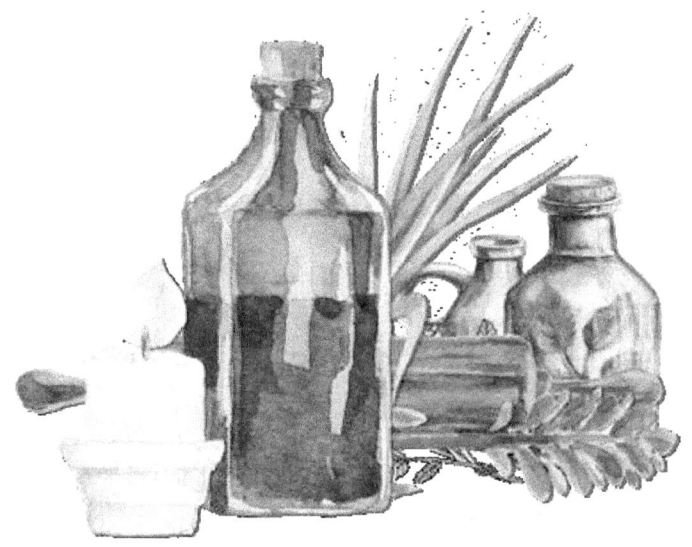

Woody, warm and herbaceous. Heart health, muscle support, emotional support. Marjoram essential oil helps to suppress or control sexual desires.

Reduces pain, eliminates spasms and cures cramps. Protects from wounds becoming septic, inhibits viral and bacterial growth, removes excess gas from intestines, cures headaches, increases perspiration, promotes digestion, increases urination, opens up obstructed menses, cures cough and cold, and dilutes phlegm. Kills fungus, lower blood pressure, cure constipation, soothe nervous disturbances, widen and relax blood vessels, improves stomach health.

Blends well with: chamomile, clary sage, cypress, lavender, myrtle, bergamot, cedarwood, eucalyptus, tea tree, and rosemary.

> *Diffuse:* *Marjoram essential oil is very effective at relieving tension with its calming properties for both body and mind and generates a happy feeling in times of anger or sadness.*

Can be helpful to calm people who have suffered a shock, trauma, or a major setback in life. Use no more than 3 or 4 drops when diffusing.

Massage: Dilute only a drop or 2 and always combine with a carrier oil to avoid irritations. of the oil on dense muscle groups after a hard workout. This will help you recover quicker and hence achieve better results at the gym.

Health: It inhibits the growth of fungus and helps cure fungal infections. This property of marjoram essential oil helps cure a number of skin diseases and other conditions like dysentery, which are all often caused by a dangerous growth of fungus.

Marjoram oil acts as a vulnerary by promoting the quick healing of wounds, both external and internal, and protecting them from infections.

This powerful essential oil helps to cure a headache, sinusitis, cold, bronchitis, asthma, stress, insomnia, pain in muscles and joints, and fatigue.

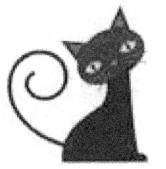 **Add your own recipe or tips here:**

MELISSA

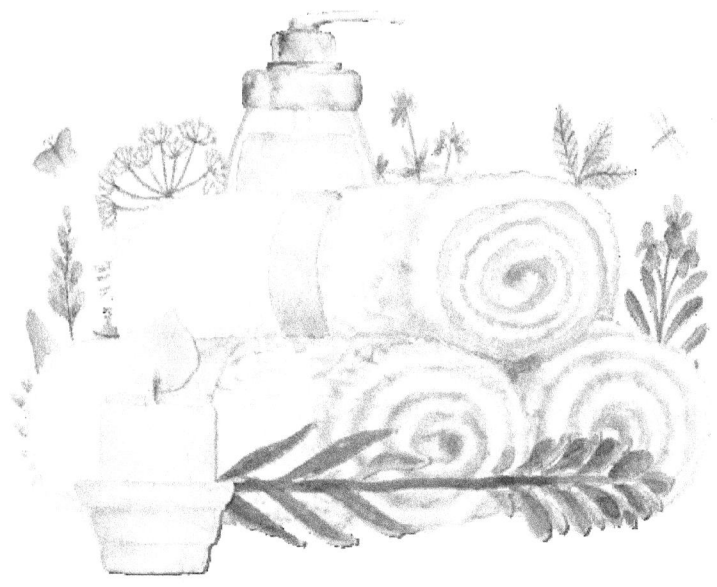

| Melissa oil is one of the rarest essential oils on the market today and provides a host of emotional and healthful benefits.

This oil has been known by several names in many cultures. It was once predominantly known as "lemon balm," but later was commonly named after the Greek word for "honey bee" because its fragrance attracted honey bees so easily.

No wonder this essential oil has earned this reputation. This is because this essential oil is extensively used in nearly all sorts of balms due to its soothing properties while having a sweet, pleasant aroma.

> *It is also known as sweet oil. Melissa essential oil is a mood lifter and an antidepressant. It has been found to inspire joy and hope. That is why it was called the "Elixir of Life" or the "Nectar of Life" all the way back in the 15th Century.*

Antidepressant, cordial, nervine, emenagogue, sedative, antispasmodic, stomachic, antibacterial, carminative, diaphoretic, febrifuge, hypotensive, sudorific, and tonic. Reduce depression, cure nervous disorders, open blocked menses, sedate inflammation, reduce spasms, inhibits bacteria, removes gas, increases perspiration & removes toxins, while reducing fever, lowering blood pressure and boosting the health of the immune system.

Blends well with: Basil oil, chamomile oil, rose oil, geranium oil, frankincense oil, lavender oil, and ylang-ylang oil.

How to use.
Diffuse: Add 3-4 drops to a diffuser.
Melissa promotes sleep, relaxes the body, and mind while bringing feelings of peace and contentment. In the past, it was used to help soldiers relax and drive away the fatigue and stress of combat.

Diffuse at night to create a calming environment and to encourage healthy and restful sleeping patterns.

To improve symptoms of dementia, diffuse melissa essential oil daily or inhale it directly from the bottle for best results.

Massage: This oil is safe to apply directly to the body without dilution. Those with sensitive skin may want to consider diluting with a carrier oil to minimize the risk of irritation.

Try blending melissa with lavender and ylang-ylang for a boost in effectiveness. Add to your bathwater for a long, relaxing soak.

Beauty: To treat skin conditions, such as eczema, use five drops per ounce of carrier oil, especially for use on the face. Alternatively, you can add 5 drops to a moisturizer or a spray bottle with water for a facial spritz.

The sedative properties makes melissa a wonderful choice for hormonal issues: irregular periods, menstrual cramps, fatigue due to periods and menopause, irritability or depression. If you are going through menopause or know someone who is, you can't go past relaxing in a hot bath with a few drops of Melissa oil added to the bath water.

Health: This oil is also found effective in the treatment of herpes, sores, ulcers, fungal infections, headaches, and fatigue. It also boosts memory. Mix 3 – 4 drops with water in a spray bottle to create a rejuvenating skin spritzer.

Promote Relaxation: 1 drop rubbed gently into the temples to ease tension from daily stress.

Nighttime Bath: An aromatic bath suffused with 4 - 5 drops of Melissa oil promotes calm, restful sleep.

Vertigo: To get rid of vertigo and nervousness, apply 2 to 3 drops topically to the back of the neck and ears to alleviate nervousness, nausea, vomiting, and dizziness.

Household: Strong antiseptic properties make this oil a great addition to homemade surface cleansers, killing bacteria and leaving behind a clean, fresh scent.

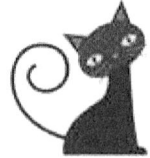

MUGWORT

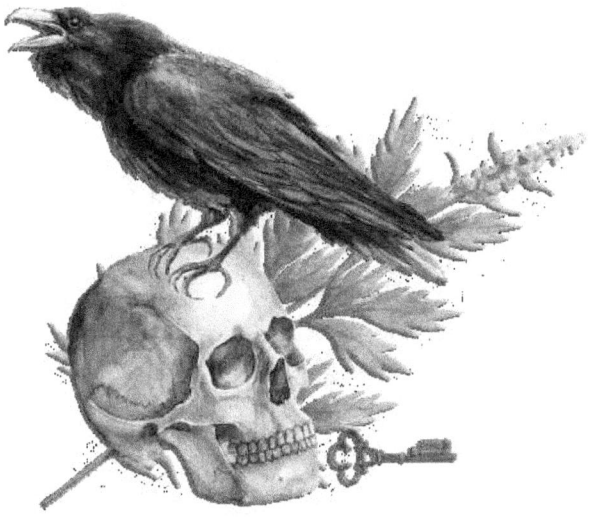

Mugwort can be considered both famous and infamous. In China, its medicinal properties were used to treat various ailments, while in European countries like England and others, it was used in witchcraft and black magic.

> *Mugwort is regarded as sacred and was associated with the supernatural and mystic forces as it was often used to prevent danger or evil spells. It was also believed to possess magical properties and to be able to increase your psychic powers!*

The essential oil of mugwort is derived from the Mugwort tree which bears the scientific name of Artemisia Vulgaris.

Cordial, digestive, diuretic, emenagogue, nervine, stimulant, uterine, and vermifuge. Facilitates digestion, increases urination and removal of toxins, treats nervous disorders, stimulates systemic functions, maintains uterine health, and kills intestinal worms.

> **Blends well with:** Cedarwood, clary sage, patchouli, cedarwood, lavender, rose, ylang ylang, juniper berry, and rosemary.

Diffuse: Helps to promote mental clarity and improve concentration levels.

Diffuse 2 drops of mugwort Essential Oil with 3 drops of lavender to promote tranquility.

To promote mental concentration and boost memory levels, blend 2 drops of mugwort oil with 2 drops of rosemary or sage essential oils in a diffuser or vaporizer and place it on your work desk table.

Add a few drops of mugwort essential oil to a herb pillow to induce dreams.

Massage: Can treat problems associated with menstruation, such as abdominal pains, fatigue, headache and even nausea.

Dilute mugwort oil with a carrier oil (coconut, jojoba or almond oil) in equal parts and gently rub it on your abdominal area.

> Dilute mugwort essential oil with a carrier oil in a 1:1 ratio, and massage it onto your lower abdominal and tummy area. Care should be taken when applying mugwort essential oil on children as it should only be used in very mild doses.

Health: Mugwort oil is also a great natural anti-epileptic and anti-hysteric remedy. It exudes soothing and calming effects on the nervous system and brain, stimulating relaxation and tranquility.

MYRRH

> *The protective witch: A protection and hex-breaking oil. Excellent for magic rituals. Anoint the house every morning and evening when needed for protection and purification.*

In ancient times, Myrrh was so valuable that it was coveted as much as gold and silver. The resin was often used in incense and perfumes in ancient Egypt.

Smoky, herbal, woody. It is a valuable addition to an aromatherapy arsenal because of its ability to work as a sedative or antidepressant.

Emotional balance, cleansing, skin health. Curb microbial growth, tighten gums and muscles and reduce hemorrhage. Alleviate coughs and colds, stops fungal growth, stimulates discharges and systems, reduces excess gas, is good for stomach health, relief from phlegm, promotes sweating, helps heal wounds quickly and protects them from infection. Protection against diseases improves circulation, and protects from rheumatism & arthritis, boosting health and immunity, sedating inflammation, and reducing spasms.

Blends well with: Bergamot, chamomile, clove, cypress, eucalyptus lemon, frankincense, geranium, grapefruit, jasmine, juniper, lavender, lemon, neroli, patchouli, rose, rosemary, sandalwood, tea tree, vetiver, and ylang ylang.

Diffuse: Diffuse 2 – 3 drops to create an aura of relaxation and calm, reducing the side effects of stress and tension and promoting a state of emotional well-being.

Myrrh oil can also be diffused when you are sick to help improve the symptoms of bronchitis, colds or coughs.

Blend myrrh with bergamot, grapefruit or lemon to help lighten up its fragrance. 2 drops of each.

Beauty: Myrrh can help maintain healthy skin. It can help soothe chapped or cracked skin.

Add 1-2 drops to a facial cleanser to harness its cleansing and astringent properties in order to promote a youthful complexion.

Health: Historically, myrrh was used to treat wounds and prevent infections. It can still be used in this manner on minor skin irritations such as athlete's foot, ringworm, and acne. Apply a few drops to a cloth before applying it directly to the skin.

Myrrh oil is used as a fungicide or antiseptic. It can help reduce fungal infections such as athlete's foot or ringworm, when applied directly to the affected area. Use on small scrapes and wounds to prevent infection.

Your recipe:

Myrrh essential oil is not recommended for those using anticoagulants such as it may have potential interactions with these medications. It is not recommended for people on diabetes medication as there is a potential for a drug interaction.

MYRTLE

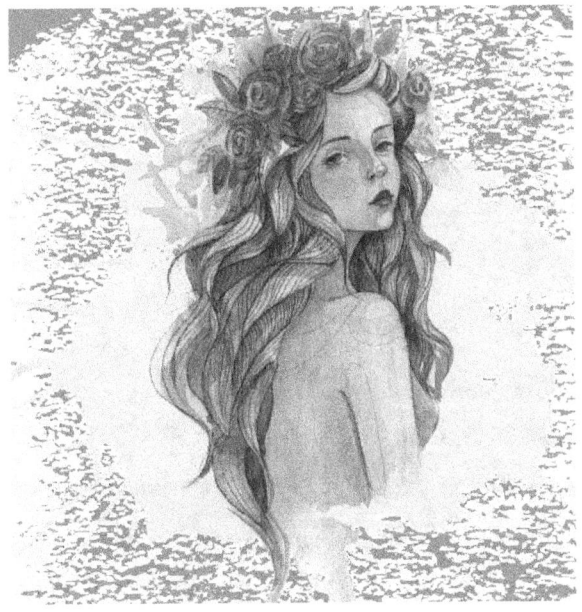

> *Myrtle is often included in weddings as a wreath or garland.*
> *During ancient times, the myrtle plant was associated with*
> *Aphrodite, the Goddess of Love and Beauty.*

Antiseptic, astringent, deodorant, expectorant, and a sedative. Increases wound healing and protects ulcers from developing more serious infections. Tightens the gums and muscles, prevents hemorrhaging, reduces body odor, fights coughs & colds and soothes inflammations. Settles nervous disorders.

Blends very well with: Clary sage, clove lavender, black pepper, rosemary, rose, and ylang-ylang.

Diffuse: Myrtle essential oil can be diffused to induce a loving and positive atmosphere - transforming sadness and grief.

Used alone or alongside of jasmine, myrtle will encourage intimacy and romance.

Blend 2 drops of Myrtle with 2 drops of rosemary and 2 drops of thyme.

Add 3 drops of myrtle oil in your diffuser with 2 drops of lavender, 2 drops of rosemary, and 2 drops during the cday to stay comfortable during the cooler months.

Myrtle encourages sleep to an active mind at bedtime. Add 2 drops to your diffuser. Myrtle allows a path for a clear calmness to create a deeply rejuvenating, restful night.

Health: If used in mouthwash, myrtle essential oil makes the gums contract and strengthen their hold on the teeth.

Myrtle essential oil works very well to alleviate problems like impotency, frigidity, erectile dysfunctions, and loss of libido.

Soak a cloth in a 4 drops of myrtle oil and very warm water. Place over chest area and cover with warm compress to calm and clear the breath.

Add 4 drops of myrtle to warm bath water before bedtime to promote relaxation and restfulness.

Household: Myrtle essential oil eliminates foul odors. It is ideal as a room freshener. Add 8 drops to a cup of water and spray inside bins.

NEROLI

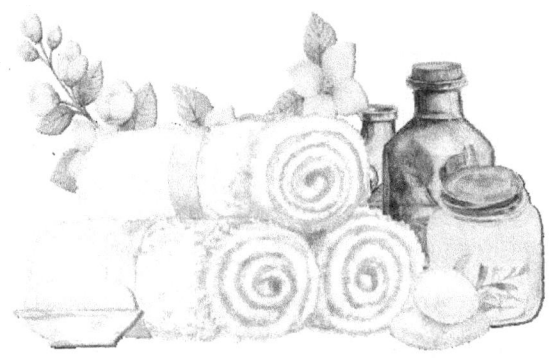

The naughty witch: *Rub between the breasts to attract men.*

Neroli oil is used in expensive colognes and perfumes and was given its name after the Countess of Nerola, an Italian Princess from the 17th century who used it to perfume her gloves and bathwater.

> *Not only does it promote arousal, it also helps fight frigidity, impotence and erectile dysfunctions. It has also been known to create romantic and sexual feelings, which is very important for having a happy and successful sex life. As they say, "Sex is in the brain!"*

Neroli Essential Oil drives away sadness, invokes a feeling of joy and happiness while uplifting your overall mood. That is why this oil is used extensively in Aromatherapy techniques.

Uplift mood and fight depression, enhance libido, protect wounds against infections, kill bacteria, relief from gas. Speeds up the fading of scars and after marks, promotes cell growth, fights infection, reduces spasms, eliminates body odor, improves digestion, takes care of skin, soothing anxiety and inflammation.

Blends well with: Chamomile, clary sage, coriander, frankincense, geranium, ginger, grapefruit, jasmine, juniper, lavender, lemon, mandarin, myrrh, orange, rose, sandalwood and ylang ylang.

How to use.

Diffuse: Diffuse neroli essential oil in your home or office to clean the air and breathe in its anti-germ properties.

Diffuse 2 drops neroli oil with 5 drops lavender to encourage deep, restful sleep and feelings of calm and tranquility.

Massage: Neroli is renowned for its ability to enhance sensual and euphoric moods.

Soothing Massage Blend: 2 drops neroli, 4 drops orange, 8 drops ginger oil, 2 drops black pepper, in 1 tablespoon of jojoba oil.

Beauty: Neroli Essential Oil works better than any anti-mark cream or lotion. The most popular properties of neroli essential oil are its ability to treat the skin. It makes the skin smooth and adds a glamorous glow. It also helps to maintain the right moisture and oil balance in the skin.

To treat breakouts. Wet a cotton ball with water, then add 3 drops of neroli oil. Dab the cotton ball on the problem area gently once a day until the blemish clears up.

Regenerate skin: Mix a drop or 2 of neroli essential oil with a teaspoon jojoba oil and apply to skin.

Health: To treat a cut, apply Neroli oil to the wound. This will effectively protect wounds from infections and tetanus.

Add 2 drops neroli to bathwater to support feelings of well-being and to soothe the skin.

> *Sweet dreams:* Put a drop of neroli essential oil on a cotton ball and place it inside your pillowcase to aid relaxation and sleep.

Soak away stress: To naturally remedy anxiety, depression, hysteria, panic, shock, and stress, add 4–5 drops of neroli essential oil to your next bath.

PMS relief: Works as a natural remedy for PMS cramps. Mix a few drops of neroli into your bathwater.

Ease labor: Childbirth - Neroli can be used to help with fear and anxiety during child labor. Diffuse it in the air, or massage it into the lower back.

Stretch marks: Add a few drops of neroli oil to your favorite cream to reduce stretch marks and broken capillaries.

Household: This essential oil can eliminate odors. It can also be used on the body as a perfume or in rooms room fresheners or vaporizers. This will not only drive away odor but will also disinfect the rooms against germs and toxins.

Homemade Neroli Body & Room Spray.

YOU'LL NEED:

1/2 cup distilled water.

22 drops neroli oil.

DIRECTIONS:

Mix oils and water in a spray bottle.

Shake well to combine.

Mist skin, clothing, curtains, and bed sheets.

ORANGE

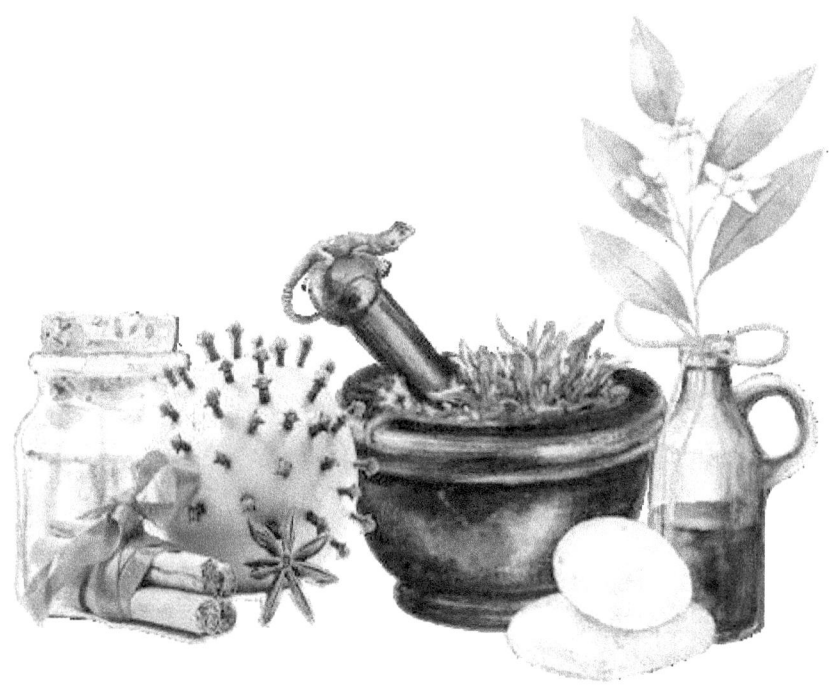

> **The seductive witch:** *Wear this oil to entice a husband or boyfriend. Add it to your daily bath to gain feelings of attractiveness.*

Well-known for its uplifting and worry-reducing properties, orange oil carries cheerfulness while simultaneously calms, making it ideal as an overall mood enhancer and relaxant. Sweet, citrusy, tangy, intense, concentrated. Emotional balance, cleansing, purifying, stimulating. Anti-Inflammatory, antidepressant, antispasmodic, antiseptic, aphrodisiac, carminative, diuretic, tonic, sedative and a cholagogue (stimulating the flow of bile from the liver). Soothe inflammation, fight depression and uplift mood, protect against sepsis, enhance libido, cure for sexual dysfunction. Relief from gas, increases urination and removes toxins, general health of the immune system, reducing emotional and nervous disturbances, increasing discharge and secretions from glands.

Blends well with: Basil, bergamot, black pepper, cinnamon, clary sage, clove, coriander, eucalyptus, frankincense, geranium, ginger, grapefruit, jasmine, juniper, lavender, lemon, marjoram, myrrh, neroli, nutmeg, patchouli, petitgrain, rose, sandalwood, vetiver , and ylang ylang.

Diffuse: Diffusing orange oil in your home, add some to your shower or perfume, or inhaling it directly from the bottle can lift your mood and bring on relaxation.

Diffuse a drop or 2 (no more than 4) to induce energizing feeling, and improving the overall scent of your home, and it's going to purify the air.

Diffuse a drop or 2 in your office for energizing your mood. This may help you get through the lethargic early hours of the afternoon.

Beauty: Before applying orange oil to your skin, dilute with a carrier oil like coconut or jojoba oil in a 1:1 ratio. Orange essential oil is also very beneficial for fighting signs of aging like wrinkles and dark spots since it promotes the production of collagen.

Combine 2 drops of orange oil with 2 drops of frankincense oil, 2 drops of geranium oil to a teaspoon of coconut oil, then massage into skin.

Health: Orange oil can fight microbial growth, protecting teeth and gums from harmful infections. It has also been used to help ease a sore throat for fast relief when gargled with water and salt. You can use it to reduce cold sores and mouth ulcers when swooshing it in your mouth with water like a mouthwash.

Household:

> *Garden Insect Spray: 4 drops orange oil, 2 drops grapefruit oil, 2 drops lavender oil, 2 drops chamomile oil in 4 oz bottle; spray affected leaves.*

Kitchen Cleaner.

Orange oil has a natural fresh, sweet, citrus smell. Diluted, it's a great way to clean countertops, cutting boards or appliances without needing to use bleach or harsh chemicals.

Add a few drops to a spray bottle with other cleansing oils like bergamot oil, water, and a small amount of coconut oil before using all throughout your home.

Deodorize your dishwasher by combining orange oil and 1 cup of lemon juice (freshly squeezed if possible). Add to the bottom of your dishwasher and run the rinse cycle only to disinfect and deodorize. You can use the same formula to clean the kitchen sink.

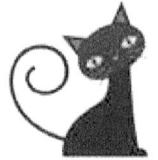 **Add your own recipe here:**

OREGANO

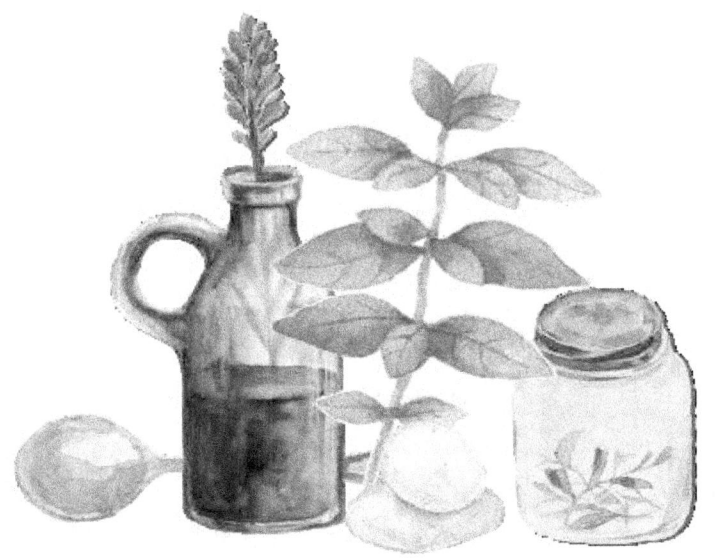

| *These blooms are so delicious and attractive to bees that it is recommended to plant them in pollinator gardens to attract bees and butterflies.*

Oregano is a plant native to higher altitudes and typically grows in the mountains, which is how it is named "Oregano," meaning "delight of the mountains."

Warm, spicy-herbaceous, and camphoraceous. Healthy digestion, respiratory problems, powerful cleansing agent. Antiviral, antibacterial, antifungal, anti-parasitic, antioxidant, anti-inflammatory, digestive, emenagogue, and an anti-allergenic. Inhibits viral, bacterial, fungal, and parasitic infections. Soothes inflammations, promotes digestion, opens up obstructed menstruation, helps cure allergies.

Blends well with: Bergamot, cedarwood, chamomile, cypress, eucalyptus, lavender, lemon, orange, rosemary, tea tree, and thyme.

Diffuse: When diffusing, 3 or 4 drops will do the job.

It can be diffused on its own, but due to its strong herbaceous scent, it is often recommended to pair it with other oils. It works best in a blend. When blending with other oils, reduce the drops used.

When diffused, oregano is employed to boost immune function, especially during the cold and flu season, and to support respiratory function to help ease mucus production.

Massage: 1 or 2 drops in a carrier oil are all you need for a massage.

Ideal for toenail and fingernail fungi.

Health: Add one drop to a glass of water and swish in the mouth (but do not swallow) for gum and tooth health.

Oregano oil is beneficial for regulating menstruation and delaying the onset of menopause. Those suffering from obstructed menses may also find relief by using oregano essential oil. As an emmenagogue, it can help a woman reduce her symptoms of oncoming menopause, including mood imbalance and hormonal shifts.

Household:

> *Create an inexpensive cleaner.* Add 10 drops to 2 cups of water in a spray bottle for a quick and easy surface cleaner. The purifying properties and the tangy scent will help your kitchen look and smell cleaner.

PATCHOULI

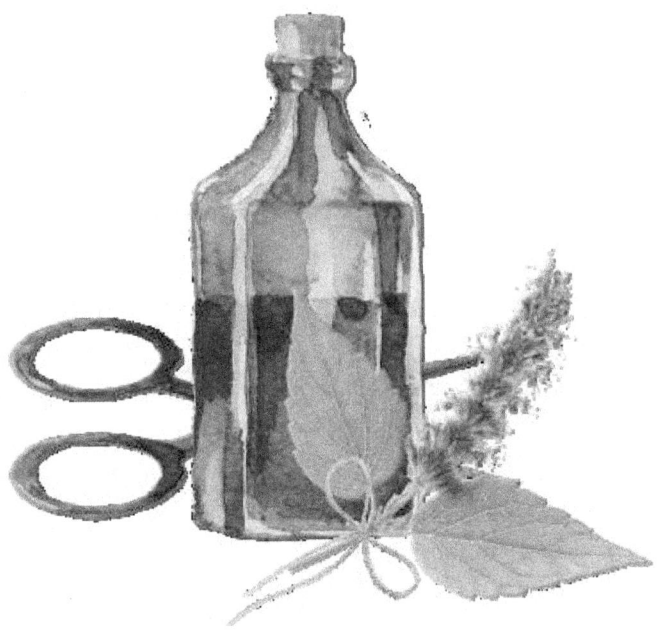

> **The sensual witch:** *A powerful oil to attract women. Also wards off negativity and evil, gives peace of mind, and is very sensual.*

The insecticidal and insect repellent properties of patchouli oil have been known for many years, particularly as it was used in the protection of clothes and fabrics from insects. Herbal, musky, sweet.

Patchouli oil is also useful for treating sexual problems including impotence, loss of libido, disinterest in sex, erectile dysfunctions, frigidity, and sexual anxiety. Patchouli oil has been used as an aphrodisiac for hundreds of years.

Healthy skin, complexion, tension, stress, grounding. Soothes inflammation from high fevers, inhibits wounds becoming septic, increases libido, cures sexual disorders. Helps tighten gums and muscles, stops hemorrhaging, heals scars and after marks, promotes cell growth, eliminates body odor, increases urination and removes toxins. Cure fever, kill fungus and insects, reduce emotional and nervous disorders.

Blends well with: Bergamot, black pepper, cedarwood, chamomile, clary sage, clove, cinnamon, coriander, frankincense, geranium, ginger, grapefruit, jasmine, lavender, lemongrass, mandarin, myrrh, neroli, orange, rose, sandalwood, and vetiver.

Diffuse: Inhalation can stimulate the release of happy hormones such as dopamine and serotonin, which can dispel feelings of anxiety and sadness to promote a balanced emotional state.

Diffuse 3-4 to encourage calm and peace, promoting healthy, restful sleep.

Uplifting blend: Combine 2 drops of patchouli with 2 drops of ylang-ylang, 2 drops of bergamot and 2 drops of frankincense.

Massage: Combine 2 drops patchouli with 2 drops peppermint oil in a teaspoon of carrier oil and massage into neck and temples to relieve stress.

Beauty: Add 1-2 drops to a facial moisturizer or cleanser to promote smooth, healthy skin and may reduce the appearance of blemishes, fine lines, wrinkles, and skin spots.

It is also used in a carrier oil to apply to **nails** suffering from yellowing or cracking.

Hair: Massage 5 drops of patchouli oil into your scalp or add it to your conditioner.

Personal deodorant: Rub 1–2 drops under your armpits or add it to your favorite body lotion.

Health: Patchouli essential oil helps to quicken the healing process of cuts and wounds, and also hastens the fading of scars. It is similarly effective in eliminating marks left by boils, acne, pox, and measles.

Topical application can fight fungal growth and infections.

> *Aromatic Bath: Add 10 drops of patchouli oil to a relaxing bath to feel deeply moisturized and nourished.*

To speed up the healing process of unwanted marks on the skin, rub 2–3 drops of patchouli oil into your hands and then apply it the scarred area.

Household: Despite smelling sweet, it is very effective at keeping insects at a distance. Mix with water to wash clothes and bed linen to deter mosquitoes, ants, bed bugs, lice, fleas, flies, and moths.

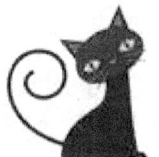 **Add your own recipes and tips here:**

PEPPERMINT

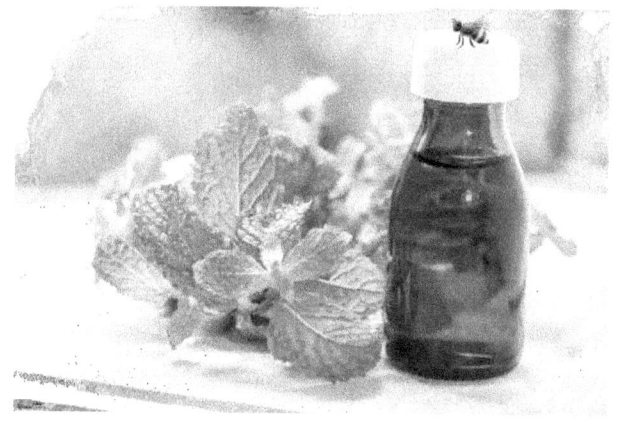

The financial witch: Used to create financial gains within one's life. Also used to relax and allow one to unwind.

Most recognize peppermint as an ingredient in toothpaste and mouthwashes, but this herb has the honor of being one of the world's oldest medicines.

Not only is peppermint one of the oldest herbs used for medicinal purposes, other historical accounts date its use to ancient Chinese and Japanese folk medicine. It's also mentioned in Greek mythology the nymph Mentha was transformed into an herb by Pluto who had fallen in love with her and wanted people to appreciate her for years to come.

The health benefits of peppermint oil as well as peppermint oil uses have been documented back to 1,000 BC and have been found in several Egyptian pyramids.

Cooling, energy, digestive and respiratory support. Pain relief - induce numbness, protect against sepsis, reduce milk flow and discharge, relax spasm, strengthen gums, stop hair loss, lifts skin. Produces firmness in muscles, stops hemorrhaging, removes gas, brain and memory health, promotes bile discharge, clears congestion and eases breathing. Relieves obstructed menstruation, expels phlegm & catarrh, reduces fever, is good for liver, and stomach.

How to use.

Diffuse: Add 3-4 drops to a diffuser.

The invigorating, refreshing, cooling and reassuring aroma of Peppermint essential oil boost mental power. The oil also helps in enhancing your mental strength, treating stress, reducing fatigue and anxiety. It also helps in managing anger, mental strain, confusion, nervousness, palpitations, vertigo, and depression.

Inhaling peppermint essential oil during mealtimes to help you feel full faster.

> *Peppermint will perk you up during long road trips, in school, or any other time you need to "burn the midnight oil."*

Diffusing peppermint along with clove oil and eucalyptus oil can also reduce allergy symptoms.

Beauty: Peppermint oil contains menthol, which is good for the skin because it gives a cooling sensation. Furthermore, it nourishes dull skin and improves the texture of oily or greasy skin.

Add 2-3 drops of peppermint essential oil to your morning shampoo and conditioner to stimulate the scalp, energize your mind, and wake you up!

Because peppermint is a powerful antiseptic, peppermint can also help remove dandruff and lice.

> *This oil can be topically applied to the nails to reduce the risk of fungal infections.*

Massage: Add several drops to massage oil or lotion to cool skin after being in the sun.

After-a-workout Blend: 5 drops ginger oil, 6 drops peppermint oil, 6 drops Eucalyptus oil in a tablespoon of carrier oil, massage into muscles and joints.

Soothing Belly Blend: 4 drops grapefruit oil, 4 drops peppermint oil, 2 drops ginger oil, 2 drops fennel oil in a tablespoon of carrier oil.

Health: Peppermint oil aids in treating eczema, lesions, acne, insect bites, rashes, allergies, irritation, and itchiness.

> *Anti-Itch: To soothe poison ivy, apply some peppermint oil mixed with lavender oil to soothe the itch.*

Teething -Peppermint oil is a natural remedy to relieve the pain associated with teething in infants. Mix peppermint oil with coconut oil at a 1:1 ratio and rub on the gum area.

Mouthwash: Combine a drop along with a drop of lemon oil in a glass of water to make a refreshing mouth rinse.

> **Household:** *Natural Bug Repellant –Ticks aren't the only bugs that hate peppermint oil. Ants, spiders, cockroaches, mosquitos, mice, and lice are repelled by peppermint.*

ROSE

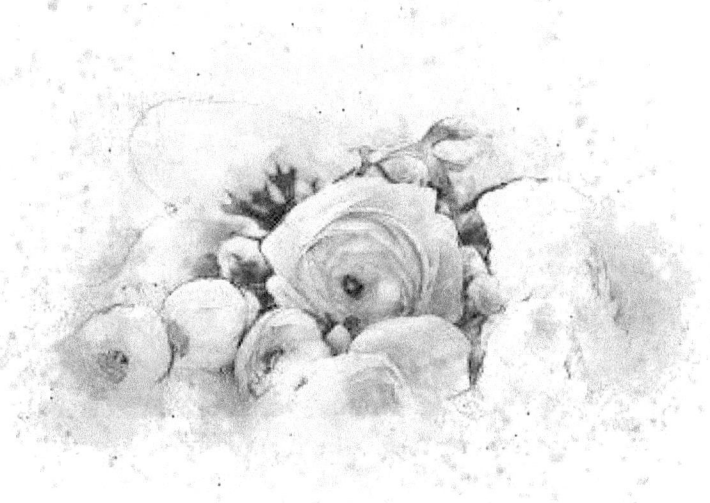

> **The loving witch:** Used in all love spells and rituals to induce peace and harmony. The smell of a rose invokes fond memories of young love and backyard gardens.

Emotional balance, clear skin, complexion. Fight depression, uplifts mood, soothes inflammation due to fever, protects wounds against developing sepsis, relieves spasms, fights viral infections, enhances libido, cures sexual disorders, tightening gums and muscles, stopping hemorrhaging. Inhibits bacterial growth, promotes discharges and secretions, heals scars, purifies the blood, opens up obstructed menses, stops hemorrhaging, boosts liver health, cures constipation and nervous disorders, stomach and uterine health.

Blends well with: Bergamot, Chamomile German, Chamomile Roman, Clary Sage, Geranium, Melissa, Rosewood, Sandalwood and Ylang-ylang.

Diffuse: If you're feeling anxious or down in the dumps, try putting 5 drops of rose and 5 drops of lavender in a diffuser by your nightstand before bed.

> *Massage: Combine 4 drops of rose, 4 drops of sandalwood, 4 drops of jasmine, and 4 drops of Ylang-ylang with 2 tablespoons of coconut oil for a romantic massage for two.*

Beauty: Acne: try dabbing one drop of pure rose essential oil on blemishes three times a day. For delicate skin, dilute with equal parts coconut oil.

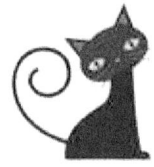 **Add your own recipes and tips here:**

ROSEMARY

"There's rosemary, that's for remembrance, pray you love, remember." ~ Ophelia

(Shakespeare's "Hamlet")

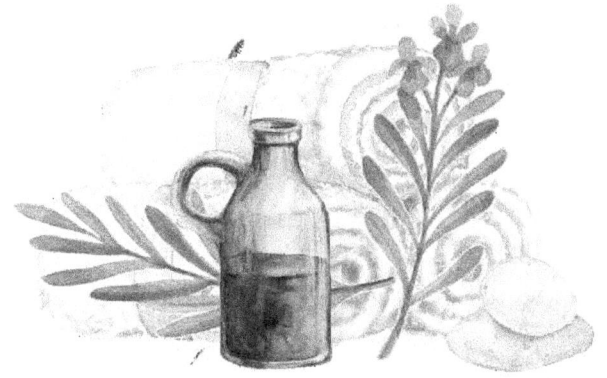

> *The self-assured witch:* Rosemary is used in healing rituals, and to promote prudence, common sense, and self-assurance. It aids mental powers and is ideal for protective spells and talismans.

Rosemary has long been used for rites of passage and to symbolize love, remembrance, trust, and friendship. The Greek and Romans made rosemary garlands and headdresses for weddings and celebrations and burned rosemary incense at funerals. Rosemary is thought to bring good luck and to impart protection and was one of the original ingredients in "Four Thieves" or "Marseille" vinegar, used by bandits to protect themselves in medieval times from the plague. Up until recently, many French hospitals used rosemary to disinfect the air.

Rosemary oil is an excellent brain and nerve tonic. It is often used by students during exams because it increases concentration and helps in studying efficiently. It stimulates mental activity and is remedy for depression, mental fatigue, and forgetfulness. Inhaling rosemary oil seems to lift your spirits immediately. Whenever your brain is tired, try inhaling a little rosemary oil to remove boredom and renew your mental energy.

Respiratory support, memory, digestion, healthy hair/scalp. Stimulating hair growth, disinfectant, antiseptic, anti-inflammatory, antibacterial, depression, carminative, and analgesic substance. Hair care, skin care, oral care, anxiety, mental disorders, pain, headache, rheumatism, respiratory problems, bronchial asthma, indigestion, and flatulence.

Blends well with: Basil, Bergamot, Cedarwood, Frankincense, Ginger, Lemon, Orange, and Peppermint.

Diffuse: Diffuse rosemary oil when you're in need of a clear mind and a boost of warming energy. Works quickly to refresh a dull and hazy mind and to promote clarity and inspiration for creative projects.

Give it a try with 4 drops of orange or with your favorite citrus for a bright and uplifting result.

Mental Clarity Inhalation Blend: 8 drops rosemary oil, 4 drops peppermint oil and 4 drops lemon oil.

Massage: For a tired and overworked body, dilute 10 drops of rosemary in a tablespoon of carrier oil and gently massage into affected areas, or add to a warm bath for a long soak.

Deep Breath: 8 drops frankincense oil, 6 drops eucalyptus oil, 3 drops rosemary oil, and 3 drops peppermint with 2 tablespoons of jojoba oil. Rub on chest. Alternately, add oils to a warm bath.

Improve Memory: Mix 3 drops of rosemary oil with 1/2 tsp of coconut oil and rub on upper neck.

Reduce Pain: Mix 2 drops of rosemary oil, 2 drops of peppermint oil, and 1 tsp of coconut oil - rub on sore muscles and painful joints.

Beauty: Hair: Mix 20 drops of rosemary oil into a cup of water and rub the mixture onto your scalp and on your hair strands. This is believed to be able to slow graying, stop dandruff, increase growth, and keep the scalp free of irritation or infection.

Hair and Scalp Formula: 8 drops rosemary oil, 4 drops cedarwood, 4 drops lemongrass, 4 drops peppermint, and 4 drops lavender in 2 tablespoons of jojoba oil.

Household: When the oil is inhaled, it is known to boost mental energy and clear the respiratory tract. Many people use a mixture of rosemary essential oil and water as an air freshener to remove bad odor from the house.

Rosemary oil is also known to be a very strong natural insect repellant. Add a few drops (at least 10) to a spray bottle of water to keep insects at bay.

How to make Rosemary Oil.

Make Rosemary oil at home with a simple recipe. Removing the rosemary from the stem until you have at least 1 cup. Next, heat 2 cups of sunflower oil in a slow cooker along with the needles. Set it at a low heat for 5-6 hours; you will start to smell what the final product will be. Let the oil cool then strain the needles out. Done!

Notes:

SAGE

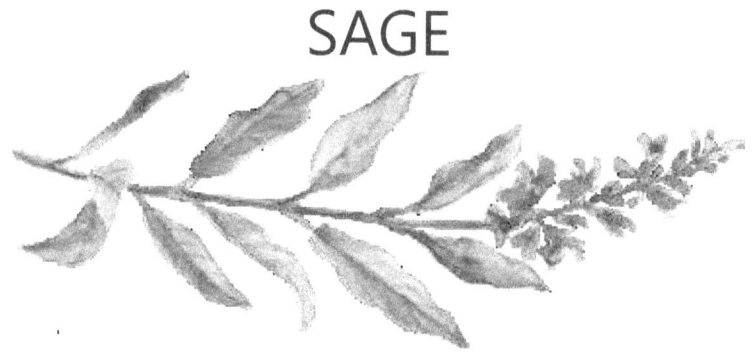

> *Sage gets its name from the Latin word "salvere," which means "to save."*

This oil is often compared to clary sage (Salvia sclarea). While they both come from the same family, they are very different from each other. Both oils have a pale yellow-green color, but sage has a strong, spicy scent, while clary sage has a sweet, nutty aroma. Because sage oil may trigger sensitizations in some, clary sage oil is often used as a substitute to it because of its milder nature.

Fights infections, opens obstructed menstruation, cures coughs and colds, reduces fever, helps clear the bowels, stimulates discharges, boosts systemic functions.

Blends well with: Juniper oil; geranium oil, lavender oil, jasmine oil, neroli oil; lemon oil, bergamot oil, and other citrus oils; frankincense oil, cedarwood oil, and sandalwood oil.

Diffuse: Diffuse white sage whenever negative energy needs to be cleared, and positive energy needs to be invited in. Sage is often bundled into a wand or smudge stick then burned. Today, many Native Americans use the stems and leaves for smudging, a ritual which has adopted as a modern practice by people all over the world.

Massage: Use as a massage oil or diluted in your bath water to help relax muscles. It can even help women cope with menstrual problems.

Beauty: Sage slows down aging and prevents symptoms like wrinkles, sagging skin, and muscles.

> *Health: People who drink alcohol should avoid using sage oil, as it can heighten their intoxication.*

Since it has antimicrobial, antibacterial, and antifungal properties, it serves as an antiseptic for wounds, surgical incisions, postnatal injuries, ulcers, and sores. Sage oil is equally useful at countering bacterial infections since it kills bacteria and inhibits their growth in the body.

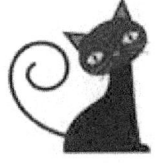 Add your own recipes and tips here:

SANDALWOOD

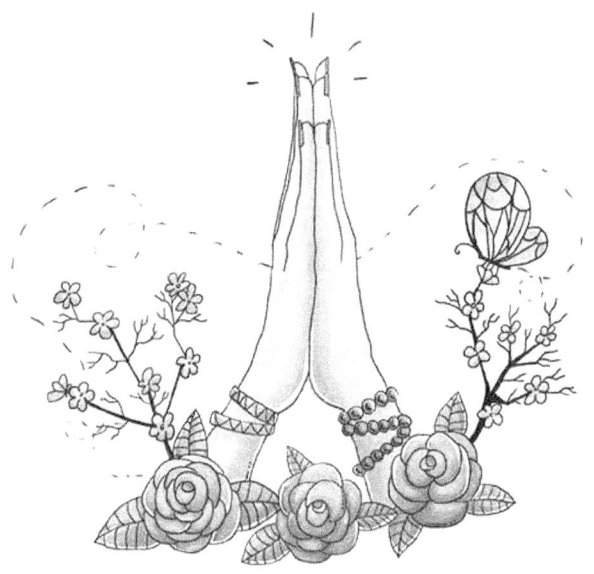

The incarnated witch: Protective and healing. Also aids in seeing past incarnations.

Sandalwood essential oil has been a part of religious practices in India along with other Eastern countries for many years. The sandalwood tree is considered holy and used for various religious ceremonies including decorations for weddings or for the birth of a baby. The highest quality sandalwood is the Indian variety, known as Santalum album. Hawaii and Australia also produce sandalwood, but it is not considered to be of the same quality and purity as the Indian variety.

About Australian Sandalwood Essential Oil: The oil from this unique species of sandalwood, Santalum spicatum, represents one of the rare success stories of the preservation of this endangered aromatic treasure. Harvesting of this variety of sandalwood is performed only under stringent license conditions enforced by the State Government, which requires that 12 seedlings are planted to replace each harvested tree.

Woody, smooth, rich, earthy, nutty, sweet. Calming, grounding, skin health. Protects wounds from infection, soothes inflammations due to fever, clears up spasms, tightens gums and muscles, stop hair loss. Reduce the chance of hemorrhage, heal scars and after marks, relief from gas, increase urination, and keeps skin smooth & free from infections. Cures coughs and colds, reduces blood pressure, improves memory, soothes nervous disorders and inflammations, and boosts the immune system.

Blends well with: Bergamot, black pepper, geranium, lavender, myrrh, rose, vetiver, neroli, and ylang-ylang.

Diffuse: Not only is sandalwood beneficial for mental clarity, it also helps to create a feeling of relaxation and peace. Since one of sandalwood's benefits is clarity, it also can work as a memory booster.

> *Diffuse 5 drops of sandalwood essential oil. Inhaling a couple of drops of sandalwood from the palms of your hands on a regular basis may induce a calming sensation. It's the perfect way to relieve some stress throughout the busy working day.*

If you are having a stressful day, diffuse up to 3 drops of the oil in your office, and this will promote the feeling of relaxation and comfort.

Wonderful diffused around children when it is time for quiet and calm.

Massage: Sandalwood is an aphrodisiac that can help increase libido, especially for men and provide energy.

Mix 4-5 drops of sandalwood with rose and vanilla oil and adding it to a carrier oil for a romantic, fragrant, woodsy blend.

Meditation Blend: 6 drops sandalwood oil, 8 drops frankincense oil, 3 drops frankincense and myrrh oil, and 3 drops cedarwood in a tablespoon of jojoba oil for topical application.

Beauty: Sandalwood oil soothes the skin, relieves it from inflammation and irritation, cures infections and keeps you feeling fresh and cool.

Add 5 drops of sandalwood oil to an unscented lotion and applying it directly to the face.

Sandalwood Perfume: Sandalwood truly is a supreme perfume. Place a drop on the wrists, neck, the crown of the head and center of the chest for a transformative effect.

Health: Applied to the skin, sandalwood reduces inflammation from mild skin irritation such as superficial wounds, pimples, warts, or boils. Apply a few drops, about 2-4, to the ankles or wrists at times of high stress or overwhelm throughout the day.

Household: Add a drop or 2 to a light bulb ring to fill the whole house with an and evoking smell.

Place 2-3 drops on the A/C vent to help maintain a calm alertness during rush hour.

Sandalwood has antiseptic properties - to help disinfect the washing machine, add 10-20 drops per load.

SPEARMINT

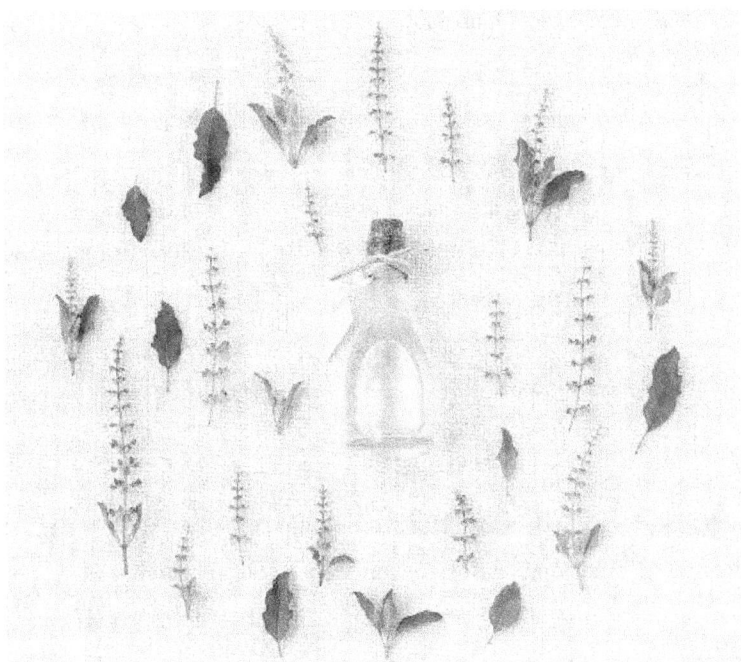

Minty, bright, sweet, pungent. Oral health, improved breath, digestive health. Antiseptic, antispasmodic, carminative, cephalic, emmenagogue, insecticide, restorative, and stimulating substance. Protect wounds from becoming septic, clears spasms, relief from gas, good for the brain, opens obstructed menses, kills insects, restores health, stimulating discharge and systemic functions.

Blends well with: Although Spearmint blends well with most essential oils, it blends particularly well with Basil, Birch, Bergamot, Eucalyptus, Jasmine, Lavender and Rosemary

Diffuse: Add 3 - 4 drops in a diffuser to clear your mind. This is great for when you are stressed out or have had a long day.

If you've been feeling sad or unhappy, inhaling the fragrance can help you feel happier and optimistic.

Massage: Mix with a carrier oil and massaged into the skin to relieve sore, hot muscles or to soothe sensitive skin.

Health: Add in a single drop to toothpaste for minty, fresh breath.

Household:

Insecticide: Spearmint oil is an effective insecticide and keeps away mosquitoes, white ants, ants, flies, and moths. It can also be safely applied to the skin for protection against mosquito bites. Spearmint essential oil is sometimes used in mosquito repellent creams, mats, and fumigants.

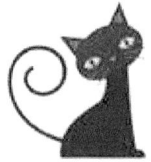 Add your own recipes and tips here:

TANGERINE

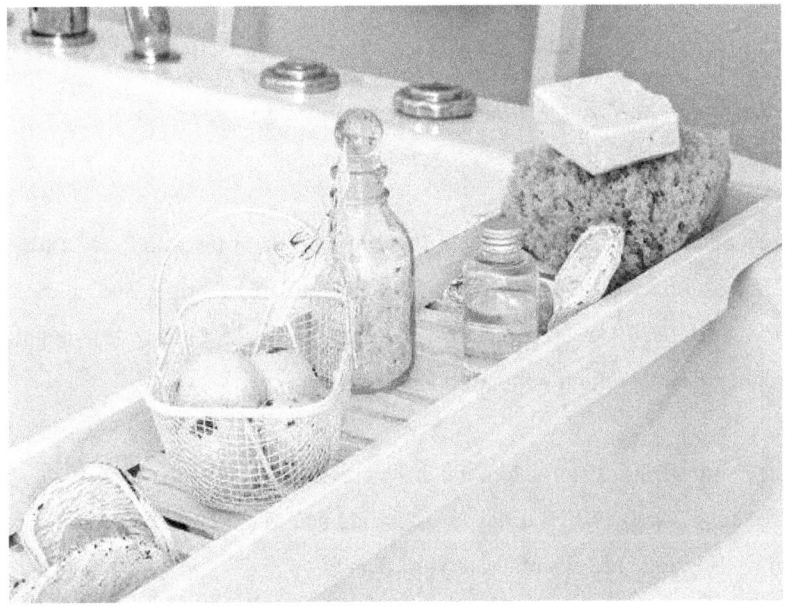

Tangerine essential oil has a long history in Chinese culture for its many health benefits in herbal medication.

It is extracted from the rind, or peel, of the fruit, and it provides numerous benefits that can be applied aromatically, topically and internally. This oil has been used to create clarity and feelings of happiness, as well as boost the immune system.

Bright, citrus, fruity. Energy, cleansing, supports the immune system. Antiseptic, antispasmodic, cytophylactic, depurative, sedative, stomachic and tonic type of substance. Protect against sepsis, relax spasms, promote growth and regeneration of cells, purifying the blood, soothing inflammation, reducing nervous disorders.

Blends well with: Bergamot, Clary Sage, Coriander, Cypress, Geranium, Grapefruit, Lavender, ginger, black pepper, and Lemon.

> **Diffuse:** *Apply 3 - 4 drops in a diffuser to energize your mind or expunge a bad mood. You may also apply 1 to 1 drops into your palms and inhale for these effects.*

To give yourself a boost of energy in the morning, or in the middle of a long day, blend it with cilantro or black pepper essential oils. The bright and spicy scents, combined with the citrus scent, will perk you up. To create a more clear-minded and happy atmosphere, blend it with lavender or ginger.

Massage: Tangerine oil is safe enough to apply directly to the skin if you avoid sensitive areas. Apply 1 to 2 drops to your abdomen to create a feeling of happiness. You may also dilute the essential oil with coconut oil.

Beauty: Helps to restore damaged skin cells and repair dark spots and scars. Combine a drop with a face or body lotion and massage into areas that have been damaged by the sun or acne.

Notes:

> **Health:** *Add a few drops to a hot bath and feel your muscles and body begin to relax.*

TARRAGON

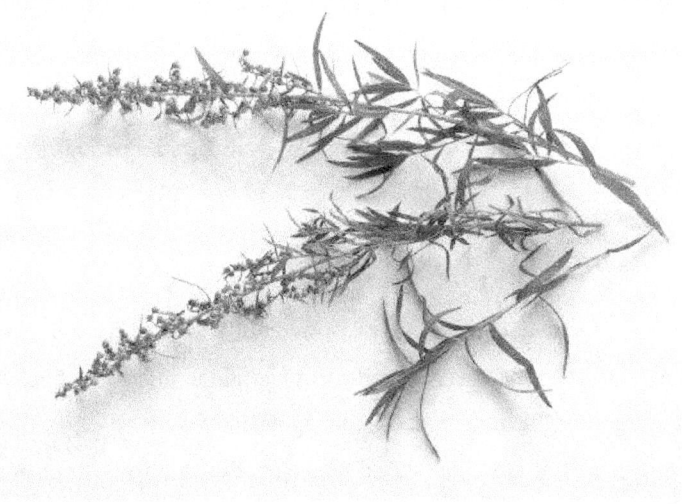

> *The name sounds strangely close to "Dragon." There is a reason for that. The common name is "Little Dragon," and the botanical name of tarragon means that as well. The botanical name for tarragon is Artemisia Dracunculus, and Dracunculus means "Little Dragon."*

Antirheumatic, aperitif, circulatory agent, digestive, deodorant, emenagogue, stimulant, and vermifuge. Treats rheumatism and arthritis, enhances appetite, improves circulation of blood and lymph, facilitates digestion, eliminates body odor, relieves obstructed menstruation, regulates the menstrual cycle, stimulates systemic functions, kills intestinal worms.

Blends well with: *Basil, carrot seed, lavender, lime, and Vanilla.*

Diffuse: Add a few drops of oil to diffusers for combating germs in the air and protecting the environment naturally.

Massage: This powerful essential oil can be diluted with carrier oils and used as a topical application or for a relaxing Ayurvedic massage.

Beauty: Add to your bathtub for an aromatic, healing, stimulating and energizing bath.

Health:

Kills Intestinal Worms: The toxicity of tarragon oil kills worms in the body. These include roundworms and tapeworms that are found in the intestines, hookworms that can live in any part of the body, and even maggots on wounds.

The spicy smell of tarragon is used to keep body odor away. It also inhibits the growth of microbes in the skin, which further reduces body odor.

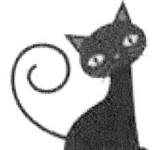 **Notes:**

> *"My love affair with nature is so deep that I am not satisfied with being a mere onlooker, or nature tourist. I crave a more real and meaningful relationship. The spicy teas and tasty delicacies I prepare from wild ingredients are the bread and wine in which I have communion and fellowship with nature, and with the Author of that nature."* — *Euell Gibbons*

TEA TREE

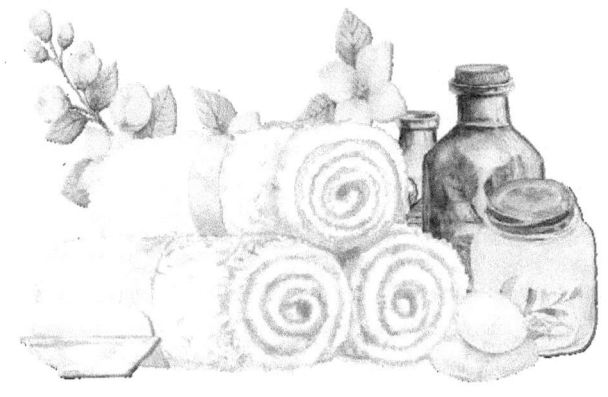

> *The magical healing and disinfectant properties make tea tree a wonderful oil that also boosts your immunity.*

It is for topical application only! Melaleuca alternifolia, or the tea tree, as it's also commonly referred to, is a plant native to the Southeast Queensland as well as the northeastern coasts of Australia and New South Wales.

Super cleansing, skin health, improves immune function. Antibacterial, antimicrobial, antiviral, insecticide, antiseptic, balsamic, cicatrisant, fungicide, expectorant, stimulant, sudorific. Inhibit bacterial, microbial, viral infections, killing insects, protecting wounds from becoming septic, promoting absorption of nutrients, speeding up the healing rate of scars. Cure cough and cold, stimulate systemic functions and appropriate discharges.

Blends well with: Geranium essential oil, clary sage essential oil, lavender essential oil, lemon essential oil, myrrh oil, rosemary essential oil, rosewood, and thyme essential oil.

Diffuse: Add 4 drops when you use it as part of your aromatherapy sessions.

Diffuse tea tree alone or in combination with eucalyptus essential oil and lavender oil, especially when colds and flu are being passed around.

Diffusing tea tree oil into the air around your home to kill mold and other harmful bacteria.

Massage: Dilute tea tree oil with a carrier oil like coconut oil in a 1:1 ratio before applying it directly to the skin.

If you are feeling tension on your back or neck, you might want to apply the oil in order to relieve the stress. You can also use it topically before and after your workout session.

Beauty: To promote healthy skin tissue, put 10 drops of tea tree oil in half a cup of water. Soak a clean cloth in the water and dab affected area.

Facial: Add 1-5 drops in a bowl of hot water and cover both the head and bowl with a towel to benefit from the healing aroma.

Scalp Health: Tea tree essential oil has significant benefits as a beneficial scalp cleanser. Pure tea tree oil can irritate the skin when applied directly, so add a few drops to your shampoo bottle.

Health: Because of its ability to kill parasites and fungal infections, tea tree oil is an excellent remedy for toenail fungus, athlete's foot and ringworm.

Put tea tree oil undiluted on the affected area using a clean cotton swab. And for stubborn fungi, consider mixing it with oregano essential oil. Tea tree oil has also been proven beneficial for treating and removing warts. Apply tea tree oil directly on the area for 30 days once or twice daily.

Tea tree oil strengthens your immunity.

Fresh Mouth: Diluted in water, pure and natural tea tree oil can be used as mouthwash.

Add 2 drops of tea tree oil to 2 oz of water - gargle.

People suffering the effects of cough and cold, congestion, bronchitis, and other associated troubles, are sure to get relief by using tea tree essential oil. Provides comfort from coughs, colds, bronchitis, and congestion. It can be rubbed on the chest and inhaled while sleeping or a drop can be placed on the pillow so it can do its magic at night and you can wake up feeling much better in the morning.

> *Insecticide: Tea tree oil is an effective insect deterrent and insect killer. It does not let parasites and other insects like mosquitoes, fleas, lice or flies come near someone who has rubbed some of this oil on their body. It kills internal insects and intestinal worms like roundworms, tapeworms, and hookworms because your body and skin can absorb it.*

Apply tea tree oil directly to wounds, boils, sores, cuts or specific eruptions, including insect bites and stings. It is as reliable as any antibiotic but without any of their adverse side effects.

For people suffering from **ear infections**, particularly children, it can be excruciating. Add a few drops of melaleuca oil into the ear to clear infection.

Thanks to the natural antibacterial nature of the oil, and it can even reduce pain and speed the healing process.

Household: Add tea tree to your household cleansers to amplify their purifying action or used directly for a more powerful effect.

Tea tree oil has powerful antimicrobial properties and can kill off harmful bacteria in the home or office. To make homemade a tea tree oil cleanser, mix with water, vinegar, and lemon essential oil then use it on your countertops, kitchen appliances, shower, toilet, and sinks.

> *Spray tea tree oil cleaner onto shower curtains, your laundry machine, dishwasher or toilet to kill off the mold.*

Add tea tree oil and lemon essential oil to your shoes and sporting gear to keep them smelling fresh!

Notes:

> *"Living is about capturing the essence of things. I go through my life every day with a vial, a vial wherein can be found precious essential oils of every kind! The priceless, fragrant oils that are the essence of my experiences, my thoughts. I walk inside a different realm from everybody else, in that I am existing in the essence of things; every time there is reason to smile, I hold out my glass vial and capture that drop of oil, that essence, and then I smile. And that is why I have smiled, and so you and I may be smiling at the same time but I am smiling because of that one drop of cherished, treasured oil that I have extracted. When I write, I find no need to memorize an idea, a plot, a sequence of things: no. I must only capture the essence of a feeling or a thought and once I have inhaled that aroma, I know that I have what I need." - C. JoyBell C.*

THYME

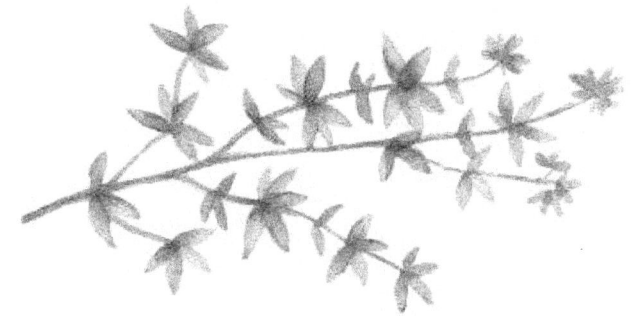

> *Thyme oil is one of the most potent antioxidants known, and it has been used as a medicinal herb since ancient times. For thousands of years, the ancient Egyptians used thyme as part of their process to assist the dead in the afterlife.*

In the middle ages, some people placed it under their pillows to purify sleep and ward off nightmares. It is botanically known as Thymus vulgaris. Eliminate spasms, relief from rheumatism by removing toxins, protect wounds from becoming septic, kills bacteria. Helps cure chest infections, coughs and colds, heart health, relief from excess gas, heals scars, increases urination, regulates menstrual cycles.

Blends well with: Bergamot, Grapefruit, Lemon, Lavender, chamomile, and Rosemary.

> *Diffuse: For diffusion merely place 3 or 4 drops in the diffuser. Thyme acts as a memory booster and an antidepressant.*

To increase circulation, diffuse 2–3 drops of thyme oil daily.

Diffuse to purify the air and maintain a sense of alertness during the day. This also is a great way to distribute antioxidants. When used outside it can help repel insects.

Massage: To relieve menstrual cramps, rub 2 drops of thyme oil with equal parts carrier oil on your abdomen.

For immune support and muscular and joint health, mix 1 drop of thyme with a few drops of lavender oil and chamomile oil in a carrier oil. Massage into skin as needed.

Health: Thyme oil kills infections, reduces anxiety, rids the body of toxins, and treat insomnia without drugs, making thyme the natural remedy for the common cold. The best part is it's all natural and doesn't contain the chemicals that can be found in medications.

To ease fatigue, add 2 drops of thyme oil to warm bath water.

To kill toe fungus, add 5 drops of thyme oil to a warm foot bath.

> *Household: It can be used efficiently to keep away parasites that feed on the human body like mosquitoes, fleas, lice, bed-bugs, and flies, as well as insects that attack food grains and clothes like beetles and moths.*

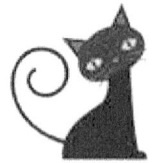

VANILLA

> **The energizing witch:** *A vitalizing oil. Also sexually arousing in women and used to restore energy.*

Madagascar is known to produce the world's finest vanilla. Neutralize the effects of free radicals and other oxidants, repairs damages due to oxidation, enhancing the libido, promoting sexual arousal. Inhibits the growth of cancerous cells, reduces a fever, fights depression, uplifts mood, soothes inflammation, reduces nervous disorders, improves sleep, and reduces stress and anxiety.

Blends well with: Rose, jasmine, ylang-ylang, bergamot, frankincense, sandalwood, orange, lemon, neroli, chamomile, and vetiver.

Diffuse: Vanillin hydroxybenzaldehyde, a component of vanilla essential oil, is a useful antidepressant and mood lifter. Vanilla is valuable in awakening passion and uplifting the mind.

Vanilla essential oil aids with a good night's sleep by lowering blood pressure, it has a tranquilizing effect on the brain.

Massage: Relax your body and mind. Massage equal parts of vanilla oil and a carrier oil and rub into your neck, feet, chest, and stomach. This relieves muscle aches, PMS cramps, feelings of anxiety and works as an antibacterial agent.

Beauty: DIY perfume, add 10–20 drops to a spray bottle and mix it with an equal part of carrier oil (like jojoba or almond oil) and water.

Romantic Perfume: 8 drops vanilla, 4 drops sandalwood, 2 drops rose in 2 teaspoons of your favorite carrier oil to create a perfume.

Health: To improve sleeping patterns, add 5–10 drops to your warm bath water.

Aphrodisiac: An administration of vanilla essential oil to patients suffering from impotence, erectile dysfunction, frigidity or loss of libido can relieve them of these problems. Vanilla essential oil stimulates the secretion of certain hormones like testosterone and estrogen which help to bring about healthy sexual behavior and promotes sexual arousal.

Household: Add 10–20 drops to a spray bottle and mix it with equal parts carrier oil (like jojoba or almond oil) and water and spray on your sheets, furniture, body, and hair.

VETIVER

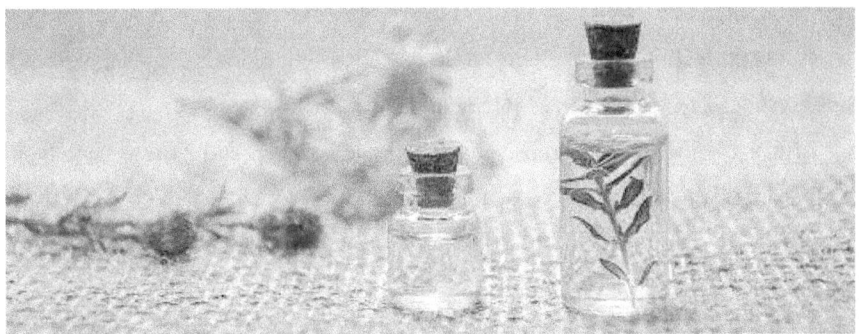

Vetiver oil, also known as khus oil, is believed to be grounding, calming, stabilizing, and provides a range of uses and benefits. Its calming and soothing properties are said to dispel anger, hysteria, and irritability, and reduce neurotic behavior.

> *Vetiver is perhaps the premier perfume fixative and is said to be a component in 90% of all perfumes.*

Caramel, sweet, smoky and woody. Anti-inflammatory, antiseptic, aphrodisiac, cicatrisant, nervine, sedative, tonic and a vulnerary compound. Soothe inflammation, protect against sepsis, enhance the libido, speed the healing process of scars and spots, cure nervous disorders, boost the body's ability to heal itself.

Blends well with: Ylang-ylang, sandalwood, clary sage, patchouli, jasmine, angelica, and lavender.

> *Diffuse:* Mix 3 drops vetiver oil, 6 drops chamomile oil, and 6 drops bergamot oil for a calming and grounding effect on your emotions.

Massage: Relaxing Body, Mind, and Spirit: Mix 3 drops vetiver oil, 6 drops chamomile oil, and 6 drops bergamot oil to your favorite massage oil.

Rest and Rejuvenation Blend: 8 drops vetiver oil, 8 drops clary sage oil and 8 drops lavender in 1 tablespoon of jojoba oil.

Injury blend: Blend 4 drops vetiver, 3 drops lavender and 2 drops bergamot in 2 Tbsp. carrier oil. Massage into the affected area.

Arthritis blend: Blend 4drops frankincense, 3 drops marjoram and 2 drops each rosemary and vetiver in 2 Tbsp. carrier oil. Massage into the affected area.

> *Beauty:* Too much sun? Add 2 drops of vetiver oil to tepid bath water and soak, or apply (diluted) onto skin for a cooling effect.

Health: Dissolve a few drops of the oil in your warm bath to ensure deep relaxation - benefits for your overall body.

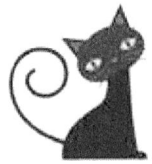 **Add your own recipes and tips here:**

WILD ORANGE

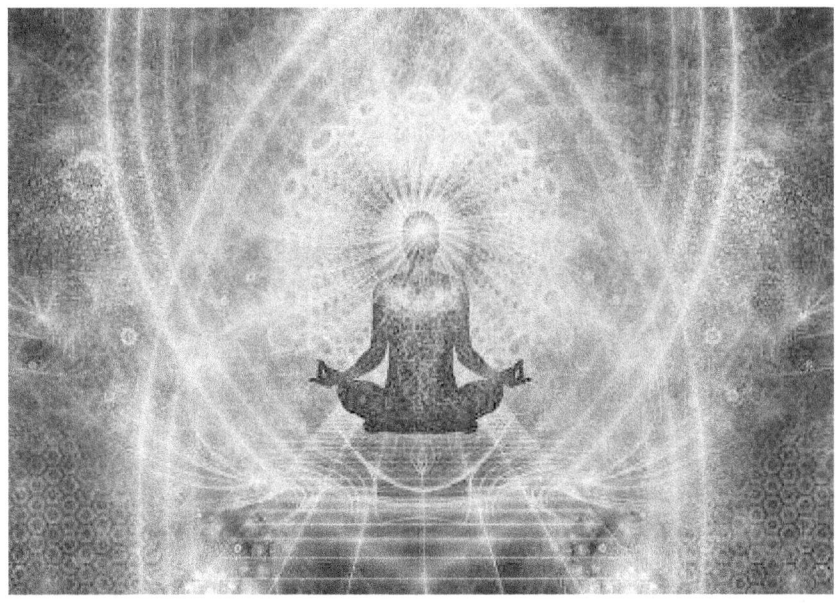

> *Due to its high measurements of antioxidants, wild orange essential oil is a great immune system booster!*

Fresh, sweet and citrus. Energy, emotional balance, overall health. Powerful cleanser and purifying agent. Uplifting to the mind and body.

Blends well with: Cinnamon, Frankincense, Geranium, Lavender, Lemon, Tangerine, and Bergamot essential oils.

Diffuse: You can purify your home by diffusing wild orange essential oil into the air. Or you can spray some into your car, and it can double up as a non-toxic air freshener.

Diffuse to uplift your mood and energy levels and to freshen the air.

> *Happiness Blend: 2 drops Bergamot, 2 drops Grapefruit, and 1 drop Wild Orange.*

Diffuse a drop or 2 to induce energizing sensation.

Diffuse a drop or two in the office to induce an energizing workplace. This may help you get through the lethargic hours in the afternoon.

Beauty: Revitalizing Body Scrub: Combine 1/2 cup coconut Oil, 1/2 cup brown sugar, 14 drops wild orange oil, 4 drops cinnamon oil. Store in an airtight glass container.

> **Health:** *Add a drop to a shirt collar, rub through the hair, or inhale from cupped hands in times of fear, doubt, or anxiety.*

Household: Use in an all-purpose spray to cleanse and purify surfaces.

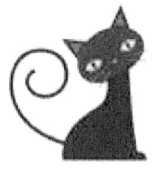 Add your own recipes and tips here:

WINTERGREEN

Wintergreen essential oil is frequently used in rubs and balms to relieve the discomfort associated with joint and muscle pain.

Emotional support, sore muscles or joints, skin health. Analgesic, anodyne, antirheumatic, antiarthritic, antispasmodic, antiseptic, aromatic, astringent, carminative, diuretic, emmenagogue, stimulating substance. Pain relief, relaxation body and mind, treatment of rheumatism and arthritis, reduction in spasms. Protects against sepsis, spreads a pleasant fragrance, tightens gums and muscles, stops hair loss.

Blends well with: Mint , oregano, thyme, vanilla, and ylang-ylang oils.

Diffuse: The strong, sweet aroma of this oil can be used to mask unpleasant odors as well as to ease tension and stress.

Diffuse 1-2 drops along with cedarwood oil in the colder months.

Massage: 1–2 drops, and mix it into coconut, olive, almond or jojoba oil before rubbing into the skin and massaging into muscles.

Homemade muscle rub - *Ideal for after a workout.*

Total Time: 20–30 minutes. Serves: 30

INGREDIENTS:

1/2 cup coconut oil.

1/4 cup grated beeswax.

2 teaspoons cayenne powder.

2 teaspoons ginger or turmeric powder.

8 drops wintergreen essential oil.

6 drops peppermint oil.

14 drops lavender oil.

Glass jar for heating.

DIRECTIONS:

Pour all oils except for the essential oils into the glass a jar.

Fill a saucepan with 2 inches of water and warm over a medium to low heat.

Place jar into the saucepan until contents melt. Stir to combine.

Add the cayenne and ginger/turmeric.

Once combined, allow to cool a little then add the essential oils. Mix well.

Pour mixture into storage containers and allow to set.

Health: *Add 1-2 drops to a bath to create a calming, warming sensation in the bath water.*

Household: Wintergreen works as a natural home deodorizer. Use wintergreen oil around your home to freshen the air and surfaces of the bathroom and kitchen. Mix several drops to water in a spray bottle - apply to hard surfaces, appliances, garbage cans and your toilet bowls.

YLANG YLANG

The irresistible witch - YLANG-YLANG: Makes its wearer irresistible to the opposite sex. Mollifies problems in married life. Worn during interviews, you will feel calmer and more in control. Sometimes called "Flower of Flowers."

The smell of ylang-ylang is unique and powerful, which is why so many perfumes and cosmetic products feature this tropical flower.

Healthy hair and skin, calming. Antidepressant, anti-seborrhoeic, antiseptic, aphrodisiac, hypotensive, nervine, sedative type of substance. Fights depression, uplifts mood, stops sebum secretion, protects against sepsis, increases libido, cures various sexual disorders, reducing blood pressure, curing nervous disorders, soothing inflammation, reducing the severity of nervous disorders.

Blends well with: Bergamot oil, grapefruit oil, sweet orange oil, neroli, lavender oil, sandalwood oil, and vetiver oil.

Diffuse: Inhaling ylang ylang can have immediate, positive effects on your mood and work like a mild, natural depression remedy. It's said to "expand the heart".

Add 3-4 drops to calm nervousness, anger, and stress.

Diffuse to use as a steamy facial to promote skin health.

For building up confidence: 2 drops ylang ylang and 2 drops bergamot.

For a natural home freshener with a tropical aroma: 2 drops ylang ylang and 2 drops jasmine.

To release tension: 2 drops ylang ylang and 2 drops frankincense.

To give you a quick energy boost: 2 drops ylang ylang and 2 drops of citrus oil like lemon oil, grapefruit essential oil or orange oil.

Massage: For an aphrodisiac massage rub: 2 drops ylang ylang and 2 drops sandalwood essential oil.

Ylang ylang is powerful at fighting the development of skin cancer cells and melanoma. Combine 1 to 2 drops with coconut or jojoba oil and massage it into the face once or twice daily for protection.

Beauty: Facial cream for combination skin: 3 drops ylang-ylang oil, 3 drops geranium oil, 2 drops rosewood oil mixed into ½ oz of your favorite facial moisturizer

Health: The loss of libido or frigidity is a growing problem in modern life, but relying on natural essential oils like ylang-ylang can really help you find your sex drive.

Add a few drops to a bubble bath to enhance feelings of relaxation and rejuvenation.

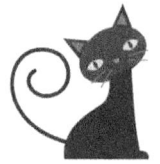 **Add your own recipes and tips here:**

POPULAR CARRIER OILS.

Carrier oils are derived from plant sources and have a neutral smell, rendering them an excellent medium for dilution and application of essential oils.

Carrier oils can vary widely in their consistency, aroma, absorption, and shelf life. Carrier oils can be blended, allowing you to mix and match until you find the blend that suits you!

Coconut Oil - Unrefined

Solid at room temperature. Distinct coconut aroma. Solid white color. Leaves a moisturizing, oily feeling layer on top of the skin. Suitable for all skin types. Absorbs relatively well and very stable with almost zero chance of rancidity. **Long shelf life.**

Fractionated Coconut Oil (Coconut oil refined)

Unlike coconut oil, fractionated coconut oil is liquid at room temperature with no noticeable aroma. Absorbs well, leaving skin feeling silky moisturized, and non-greasy. High in essential fatty acids. **Works in spray bottles, roll-ons, and doesn't stain clothes.** Processed and therefore not therapeutic. **Long shelf life.**

Grapeseed Oil

Light and thin consistency. Well suited for massages; leaves a light glossy film over the skin. Moisturizing. High in linoleic acid.

Relatively **short shelf life**

Jojoba Oil

Slightly nutty aroma. Medium consistency. Superior, non-greasy absorption, similar to the skin's natural oils. Moisturizing for skin and hair.

Long shelf life. May go rancid if not stored properly.

Olive Oil

Thicker consistency, leaving an oily feel on the skin. Stronger aroma. Good source of omega fatty acid. Has a relatively **short shelf life.**

Sweet Almond Oil *Caution: May cause a reaction to those with nut allergies.

Slightly sweet, with a nutty aroma. Medium consistency. Absorbs relatively quickly, leaving a slight hint of oil on the skin. Rich in vitamin E and oleic acid. Moisturizing.

Can stain clothes/sheets, needs to be refrigerated, and better for dry skin types

OTHER CARRIER OILS

Apricot

Rich in essential fatty acids and vitamins A and C, making this oil an excellent rejuvenating oil, especially for oiler skin. Apricot kernel oil is used as an anti-aging oil to smooth and tone the skin. Absorbs well without leaving a greasy feeling.

Has faint odor. Needs to be refrigerated and may sting dry skin.

Argan - Ideal skin moisturizer, hair conditioner, and to cure skin blemishes. Rich in antioxidants and vitamin E, Argan oil is excellent for all skin types. Has a nutty scent which may interfere with aromatherapy. Great for acne or dry skin. Very potent.

Expensive and has a distinct odor which may interfere with some essential oils.

Avocado

High in fatty acids and vitamins, avocado oil is used to increase collagen production for more youthful skin. Best when blended with other carrier oils for dry skin. Ideal for eczema. Very hydrating. Excellent for mature and very dry skin.

Doesn't absorb well into skin. Thick and heavy. Not recommended for oiler or combination skin types.

Castor oil

Castor oil stands out amongst most of the carrier oils. It contains ricinoleic acid, a rare unsaturated fatty acid that is found in high-quality cold-pressed castor oil and provides many healing benefits. Use a highgrade organic castor oil. Castor oil has a **long shelf life**. Keeping it in a refrigerator, however, is also a good idea, but more than the temperature it is the the presence of light that has a negative impact on the oil. Opaque bottles are the best choice for effective storage.

Sunflower

Sunflower oil is an inexpensive and versatile oil. Excellent oil for eczema and psoriasis. High in oleic acid and lecithin, sunflower oil is great for dry skin. Inexpensive, faint odor.

May cause breakouts for those with oily skin.

So which is the best carrier oil? Well

that depends.

I suggest trying several oils then settle on the ones you like best for your own personal needs.

TIPS ON CARRIER OILS.

For a roll-on with essential oils, use apricot, fractionated coconut, or almond oils. Make sure you store appropriately.

For a spritz in a spray bottle, use a blend of witch hazel and filtered water with your essential oils.

For a massage blend, use fractionated coconut oil as it doesn't stain fabrics.

For facials, use unrefined coconut oil, or argan with your essential oils.

For a healing mask, I like to use coconut oil blended with castor oil then add my essential oils. Castor oil has many healing powers. Such as - heals inflamed skin. Fights aging, reduces acne, moisturizes, fades blemishes, and reduces pigmentation.

Castor oil penetrates deeply into the skin and stimulates the production of collagen and elastin, keeping skin younger looking for longer while it softens and hydrates the skin. The fine lines around the eye area can also be treated with its application.

ESSENTIAL OILS - DIFFUSING BENEFITS.

A diffuser is a household must-have that can replace plug-in air fresheners to make your home smell nice. Air fresheners contain nasty chemical ingredients linked to numerous health problems. When you read the term 'fragrance' on an air freshener, it can include hundreds of toxic chemicals referred to as 'fragrance'.

If you have pets or young children living with you at home, burning candles or incense can be hazardous. With your essential oil diffuser, you can reap the benefits of aromatherapy, and to a much higher efficiency, without the risk of burns, wax spills, and other life-threatening accidents.

The term 'Diffusing' means to take a liquid and then vaporize it so that it can be inhaled and absorbed through the lungs. You receive the benefits of the oils simply by breathing as you normally would while you get on with your day. It's a simple practice, yet the benefits of using essential oils are enormous to your health and wellbeing. Essential oils not only influence your moods and increase focus and concentration, but they also support your family's immune system.

If you're a little bit witchy, then you are no stranger to natural living practices, and you probably already know a thing or two about using essential oil in diffusers to improve your health, increase your energy, and to help you sleep better. Not to mention de-stress and put you in a better mood - and who doesn't need that from time to time? I know I do. Diffusers are great for all those benefits and more. Sharing is caring, so keep one in the office to help you and your coworkers stay balanced and refreshed throughout the day. Always check with others, however. Some may not like your preferences in particular oil blends - pregnant women, for example, or those with specific allergies.

In addition to affecting our moods, inhaling essential oils can have many other benefits. Essential oils cross into the bloodstream via our lungs, quickly delivering essential oils to the whole body. Additionally, inhaling essential oils can help reduce the discomfort of respiratory infections like colds, flu and sinus congestion.

You can download my FREE Diffusing Essential Oils book now > http://amzn.to/2BLc7ZN Or buy the print book > http://amzn.to/2AxgabY

SIX POWERFUL SKIN CARE/ANTI-AGING OILS.

FRANKINCENSE - a powerful astringent, frankincense is used to help reduce acne blemishes, the appearance of large pores, wrinkle prevention, and can assist in lifting and tightening skin to naturally slow signs of aging.

MYRRH - can help maintain healthy skin. It provides relief to chapped or cracked skin and is ofen used in skin care products for its moisturizing qualities. Ancient Egyptians used this essential oil for these purposes.

SANDALWOOD - high in antioxidants, sandalwood aids in reducing damage caused by free radicals, which promote aging.

COCONUT - contains antioxidants that protect skin from damage caused by free radicals. It has anti-fungal and anti-bacterial properties which aids in healing damaged skin.

VANILLA - an excellent source of b vitamins and natural antioxidants, vanilla is a natural antioxidant which aids in protection against environmental stressors.

MANUKA – aids in healing scars and spots, promotes new growth & regeneration of cells. Filled with antibacterial properties, manuka oil aids in fighting off any bacterial growth. Bacteria is often the cause of skin conditions such as acne. Manuka Oil has wound healing properties and is used as an effective way to treat damaged skin and scarring.

Add these oils to your existing moisturizer or make your own moisturizer by adding one or a number of these oils to your preferred carrier oil, such as coconut oil, almond oil, or one of my favorites, castor oil.

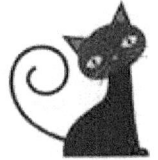 **Add your own recipes and tips here:**

SEVEN POWERFUL DESTRESS OILS.

When the scent of an essential oil is inhaled, molecules enter the nasal cavities and stimulate a firing of mental response in the limbic system of the brain. These stimulants regulate stress or calming reactions, such as breathing patterns, heart rate, production of hormones, and blood pressure. Aromatherapy can be obtained by using it in a bath, as direct inhalations, hot water vapor, vaporizer or humidifier, fan, vent, perfume, cologne, or my favorite — diffusers.

1. Lavender
2. Rose
3. Vetiver
4. Ylang Ylang
5. Bergamot
6. Chamomile
7. Frankincense

Destress blends to diffuse:

Let Go:

4 drops lavender

3 drops vetiver

3 drops ylang ylang

Field of Dreams:

2 drops ylang ylang

2 drops bergamot

2 drops lavender

Trifecta:

3 drops frankincense

3 drops lavender

3 drops bergamot

Carefree:

2 drops lavender

1 drops wild orange

2 drop geranium

1 drop clary sage

Release:

2 drops marjoram

2 drops thyme

2 drops rosemary

2 drops peppermint

3 drops lavender

Drift Away:

2 drop lavender

1 drop bergamot

1 drop patchouli

1 drop ylang ylang

Quick Lavender Neck Rub

INGREDIENTS:

6 drops pure lavender oil

2 teaspoon fractionated coconut oil or almond oil.

DIRECTIONS:

Blend the lavender oil and coconut or almond oil in your palm and rub onto your neck for natural anxiety relief. You can also rub onto the bottoms of your feet and put on a pair of socks. This is perfect for anytime or just before bed.

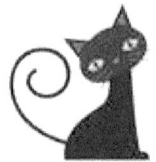 **Add your own recipes and tips here:**

ARE YOU EXPECTING?

Firstly, congratulations! You'll be very happy to know that there are lots of essential oils you can use safely during your pregnancy.

Bergamot.
Cedarwood.
Citronella* use with caution.
Clove* use with caution.
Copaiba.
Coriander.
Cypress.
Frankincense.
Geranium.
Grapefruit.
Lavender.
Lemon.
Lime.
Mandarin.
Melaleuca.
Neroli.
Orange.
Rosewood.
Patchouli.
Palmarosa.
Peppermint* use with caution.
Petitgrain.

Sandalwood.

Tangerine.

Vetiver.

Ylang Ylang.

Although Peppermint oil can assist with nausea in the early months, you should use it with caution. Peppermint oil can also help with, heartburn and other digestive upsets, however, because it is a strong oil, don't use it a lot or too often. One drop well-diluted or put in a diffuser is plenty. Using Peppermint oil past twenty-five weeks can reduce breast milk production in some women.

Lemon or Citrus Fresh oils diluted in a carrier oil and massaged into the bottom of your feet may also support the digestive problems you may be experiencing. So, put your feet up and let your partner spoil you with a much-deserved foot massage.

For fatigue, oils such as Lemon and Orange as well as a little Peppermint can be invigorating. You could diffuse these oils in the morning or mid-afternoon.

If you prefer, create a spritz spray filling a -4 oz (118 ml.) bottle of distilled water with witch hazel and 5 drops of Lemon.

Fatigued? The key is plenty of good quality sleep - 8 hours if possible. Drink plenty of fluids as dehydration can cause fatigue, especially if you are nursing. Drink plenty of water, broths, teas, and coconut water to hydrate.

For sleep. With pregnancy, often comes restless sleep. Are you tired during the day, but can't sleep at night? There are some excellent oils for relaxation that can be used safely during pregnancy. The best oils to use to promote restful sleep include Lavender, Chamomile, Cedarwood, Vetiver, and Tangerine. You can diffuse any combination of these before bed. Or you can dilute oils with a carrier oil and apply to the bottom of your feet. You can even make up a sleep spritz with water and spray the mist on your sheets and pillow.

For headaches, Grapefruit or Ylang Ylang oils work very well. For support and ease, add 1 drop per 1 tsp. to a carrier oil and rub into the temples, and the back of your neck and inhale. You can also add a drop of Peppermint oil.

You can and should enjoy essential oils during your pregnancy, just don't overdo it, and if you have any concerns, ask your physician or natural health practitioner.

You can find out more about essential oils for babies and children by downloading the FREE ebook > http://amzn.to/2BLc7ZN
Or buy the print book > http://amzn.to/2AxgabY

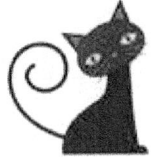 **Add your own recipes and tips here:**

RECIPES - MAKE YOUR OWN

What you'll need: some little pots to store your homemade, chemical-free, potions and lotions. Glass is always best when storing essential oils.

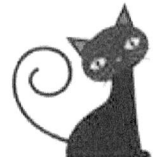 Add your own recipes and tips here:

ALOPECIA

Scalp Massage Blend.

The blend below is a 2% essential oil dilution. This means 2 drops of essential oil in 1 tsp of carrier oil. This is the recommended and safe dilution rate for adults.

With a cup of carrier oil, blend will add up to a total of 96 drops of essential oil. If your scalp is sensitive, use a 1% dilution which equals 48 drops of essential oil. Remember to do a test patch with the mixture to make sure you aren't allergic to any of the ingredients.

What you need

½ cup jojoba oil

½ cup grapeseed oil

20 drops rosemary oil

32 drops lavender oil

14 drops thyme oil

30 drops cedarwood oil

Small funnel

Amber bottle for storage

Glass dropper for application

Directions

Using the funnel, pour ½ cup of jojoba oil and ½ cup of grapeseed oil into a glass bottle.

Next, add the essential oils as directed.

Once you've added the number of drops specified, close the bottle and shake.

Your Scalp Massage Blend is ready!

How to do a Daily Scalp Massage

To use, get a glass dropper and collect some of the blend in it from the bottle. Now drop it all over your whole scalp.

Using your clean fingers, gently massage the blend into your scalp for about 4 - 5 minutes. Give particular focus, when to the bald spots.

Once your whole scalp is oiled, wash hands and cover your hair with a shower cap. This traps heat and enables the oils to penetrate deeper into the hair follicles.

Wait for about 1-2 hours then lightly rinse your hair.You can also leave without rinsing your hair.

Since this is a daily scalp massage, you don't need to wash your hair every day. Just wash it every 2 days. Use a dry shampoo to keep your hair looking non-oily.

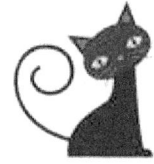 Add your own recipes and tips here:

ALLERGIES

An allergen is a trickster, making immune system think that the allergen is an invader. The immune system then overreacts to the allergen, which is basically a harmless substance, and produces Immunoglobulin E antibodies. These antibodies travel to cells that release histamine and other chemicals, causing the allergic reaction in your body.

The most common causes of an allergic reaction include:

Pollen

Dust

Mold

Insect stings

Animal dander

Food

Medications

Latex

Top 5 Essential Oils for Allergies:

Peppermint Oil

Peppermint acts as an expectorant and provides relief for allergies, as well as colds, coughs, sinusitis, asthma and bronchitis. It has the power to discharge phlegm and reduce inflammation — a leading cause of allergic reactions.

Remedy 1: Diffuse 5 drops of peppermint essential oil at home to unclog sinuses and treat a scratchy throat

Remedy 2: Apply topically to the chest, back of neck and temples. For people with sensitive skin, it is best to dilute 5 drops of peppermint with a teaspoon of coconut or jojoba oil before topical application.

Basil Oil

Basil oil helps to detoxify the body of bacteria and viruses, while fighting inflammation, pain and fatigue.

Remedy 3:

Dilute 2–3 drops of basil oil with equal parts coconut oil and apply topically to the chest, back of neck and temples.

Eucalyptus Oil

Eucalyptus contains citronellal, which has analgesic and anti-inflammatory effects. It also works as an expectorant, helping to cleanse the body of toxins and harmful microorganisms that are acting as allergens.

Remedy 4:

Diffuse 5 drops of eucalyptus at home.

Remedy 5:

Apply eucalyptus oil topically to the chest and temples – blend 5 drops with equal parts of coconut or jojoba oil.

Remedy 6:

Pour a cup of boiling water into a bowl and add 1–2 drops of eucalyptus essential oil. Placing a towel over your head, inhale deeply for 5–10 minutes.

Lemon Oil

Remedy 7:

Use lemon essential oil to disinfect your home without depending on alcohol or bleach. Lemon will remove bacteria and pollutants from your kitchen, bedroom, and bathroom — reducing the triggers inside of your home and keeping the air clean for you and your family.

Add 40 drops of lemon oil and 20 drops of tea tree oil to a 16-ounce spray bottle. Fill the bottle with pure water and a little bit of white vinegar and spray the mixture on any area in your home. Remember to spray it on your couches, sheets, curtains, and carpets.

Tea Tree Oil

This powerful oil can destroy airborne pathogens that cause allergies. Diffusing tea tree oil into the home and office will kill mold, bacteria, and fungi. It is an antiseptic agent, and it has anti-inflammatory properties. Tea tree oil can be applied to the skin to kill bacteria and microorganisms; it can also be used as a household cleaner to disinfect the home and eliminate allergens.

Remedy 9:

Add 2–3 drops to a cotton ball and gently apply to the area (rashes and hives) of concern. For those with sensitive skin, dilute tea tree with a carrier oil first, like coconut or jojoba oil.

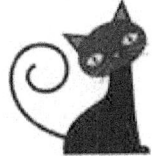 Add your own recipes and tips here:

ARTHRITIS

Pain Reliever Rub

Total Time: 2 minutes. Serves: 30

WHAT YOU NEED.

1/2 cup coconut or jojoba oil

8 drops helichrysum essential oil

12 drops lavender essential oil

DIRECTIONS:

Mix all ingredients together, then massage into painful areas.

Pour into a glass bottle and store in cool place.

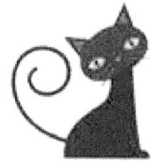 **Add your own recipes and tips here:**

ASTHMA

Clary sage: To relieve asthma symptoms, mix 4 drops of clary sage oil with 2 drops oflavender oil with a teaspoon of carrier oil and massage the blend on the chest or back.

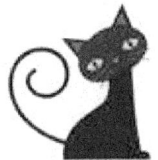 Add your own recipes and tips here:

BATHTIME

Aromatic Bath: 3 drops Roman chamomile, 3 drops lavender oil in warm bath water.

Clary sage: To improve mood and joint pain, add 3–5 drops of clary sage oil to warm bath water with 3 drops of lavender.

Cypress: Add five drops of oil to warm bath water or diffuser. It can be especially helpful to treat restlessness or symptoms of insomnia.

Fennel: Add several drops of bath water to boost strength to the body's vitality during times of sickness.

Frankincense oil immediately induces the feeling of tranquility, relaxation, and satisfaction. Add a few drops of frankincense oil to a warm bath for stress relief.

Grapefruit works as a mild, natural antidepressant while it calms the nerves. Add a few drops to your bathwater to lift your mood.

Juniper berry: To support a healthy bladder/urinary system, add a few drops to warm bath water.

Notes:

BEDTIME

Clary sage; People suffering from insomnia can find relief with clary sage essential oil. It is a natural sedative and will give you the calm and peaceful feeling necessary to fall asleep. Add 2 drops of **lavender** with 2 drops of clary sage and diffuse.

Clary sage: Sprinkle a few drops on your pillow at night for a peaceful and deep sleep.

Cypress: Add five drops of oil to your pillow or diffuse. It can be especially helpful to treat restlessness or symptoms of insomnia.

Frankincense oil immediately induces the feeling of peace, relaxation and satisfaction. Add a 3 drops of frankincense oil and 3 drops of lavender oil to your diffuser to help fight anxiety to ensure a peaceful sleep.

This all-natural night cream is great to help you fall asleep. It also doubles as a skin health-booster when applied to the skin.
INGREDIENTS:
5 drops frankincense essential oil.
5 drops lavender essential oil.
1/4 tablespoon organic coconut oil.
1/2 teaspoon castor oil.
Small container or jar to mix the ingredients.

DIRECTIONS:

Combine oils and stir together to. Massage over your face and body. May leave traces of oil on sheets.

Store to use at another time.

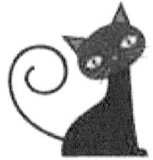

Add your own recipes and tips here:

BUG REPELLENT

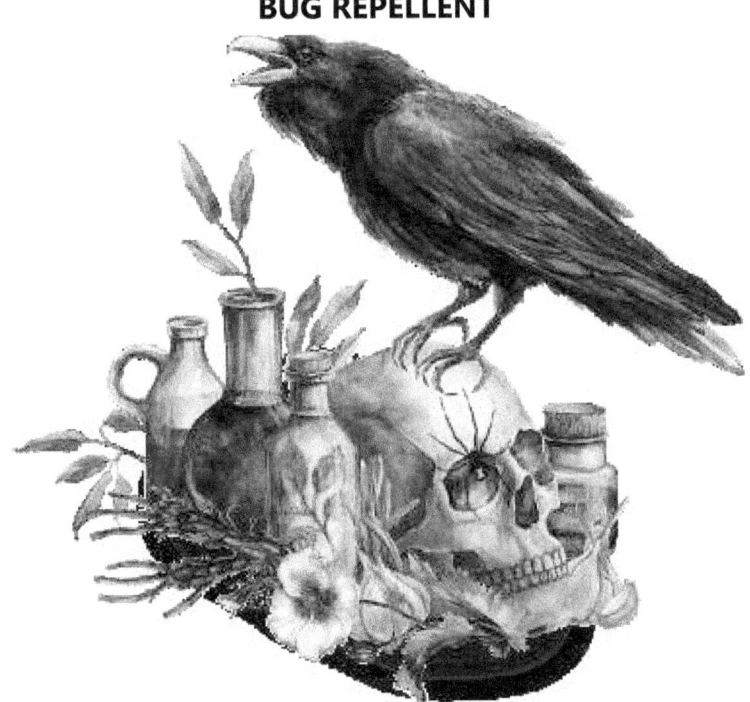

Many store-bought repellants have an unpleasant scent and contain chemicals and toxins that are harmful. Essential oils are a natural and less dangerous alternative that many believe to be more effective than aerosol repellents.

Bugger off:

1/4 cup water

3 drops clove essential oil

15 drops peppermint essential oil – kills bacteria, too.

15 drops tea tree essential oil

8 drops of citrus essential oil. Any of the following will work.

Orange

Lemon

Grapefruit.

Add drops to a spray bottle and mix with water – shake before use.

Spray problem areas on a regular basis – makes your home smell clean and fresh.

Quick bug repellant - Arborvitae: Add 8 drops of arborvitae to a spray bottle with water and spray on surfaces. Repels all sorts of insects, including moths and mosquitos. Add drops to wooded coat hangers and inside drawers to deter moths and silverfish. Can be added directly to your skin. Add to carrier oil if you have sensitive skin.

Cassia oil is useful as a mosquito repellant and works as an all-natural and chemical-free remedy. Add – 2 – 3 drops to a carrier oil and massage into skin.

Cedarwood deters mosquitoes, flies, and other insects. Sprinkled on pillows or sheets at night to ward off mosquitoes and other bugs while you sleep.

Dilute 10-20 drops with a carrier oil to make a rub on insect repellant. Carrier oils such as sweet almond or avocado oil are light on your skin and minimally greasy.

Clove oil: A few drops of clove oil placed on the bedsheets at night keep bugs away. Add a few drops to water to make a spray.

Eucalyptus oil Due to its well-known qualities as a bug repellent and natural pesticide, it is frequently used as a natural treatment for lice. Some of the mainstream treatments can be very severe and packed with dangerous chemicals you don't want absorbed into your skin. Combine a 10 drops of eucalyptus oil with enough coconut oil to massage into the scalp. Cover with a shower cap and leave for half an hour to

45 minutes before shampooing and conditioning your hair. Alternately, add a couple of drops of eucalyptus oils to your regular shampoo and conditioner.

Geranium oil is used as a natural bug repellant. To make your own bug repellent, mix 10 drops of geranium oil with ½ cup of water and spray it on your body – a much safer option than store bought sprays filled with toxic chemicals. Add baking soda to this mixture and apply to insect bites to stop itching.

Add your own recipes and tips here:

CELLULITE CREAM

Cellulite creams are often expensive and full of chemicals. Try making your own natural grapefruit cellulite. Coconut oil helps hydrate the skin, while grapefruit essential oil contains large amounts of the anti-inflammatory enzyme bromelain, which helps break down cellulite.

Total Time: 2 minutes. Serves: 30
INGREDIENTS:
30 drops grapefruit essential oil
1 cup coconut oil
glass jar.
DIRECTIONS:
Mix grapefruit essential oil and coconut oil. Store in a glass container. Rub into areas of cellulite for 5 minutes daily.

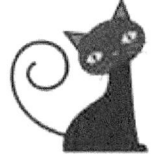

Add your own recipes and tips here:

TOP 5 OILS FOR COLD AND FLU

1. Oregano

Antiviral and antibacterial, oregano essential oil helps boost the immune system and is perfect for combating infections.

2. Thyme

With antiseptic properties, thyme can be used to stimulate circulation in those with sports injuries, pains, and strains.

3. Eucalyptus

Eucalyptus essential oil boosts the immune system while combating inflammation in the lungs. Use it to make your own steam inhalation remedy, excellent for healing sinus infections. Combine a few drops of eucalyptus oil, peppermint oil, and coconut oil for a Homemade Vapor Rub, and rub on upper chest.

4. Lime

Lime is an antiseptic, antibacterial and antiviral, meaning it will help your immune system fight off germs.

5. Frankincense

Ideal for coughs, frankincense oil is said to be a natural remedy for the lungs.

Add your own recipes and tips here:

DEODORANT

MYO Homemade Deodorant – Simplicity.

Ingredients.

1/2 cup coconut oil

1/4 cup arrowroot powder

1/4 cup baking soda

9 drops ylang ylang

8 drops frankincense

Method is the same for each deodorant.

Melt the coconut oil down into a liquid state.

Mix in essential oils.

Add in arrowroot powder and baking soda and mix until smooth.

Pour into an airtight jar or container.

Apply with your fingerstips or a small spatula.

When the coconut oil sets (this will take some time) the deodorant will be in a semi-solid state.

MYO Homemade Deodorant – Woodland.

Ingredients.

1/2 cup coconut oil

1/4 cup arrowroot powder

1/4 cup baking soda

5 drops cedarwood

5 drops geranium

4 wild orange

3 drops patchouli

Method (as above)

MYO Homemade Deodorant – Lavender dayz

Ingredients.

1/2 cup coconut oil

1/4 cup arrowroot powder

1/4 cup baking soda

10 drops lavender

4 drops lemon

3 drops rosemary

Method (as above)

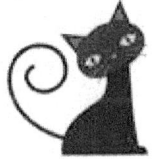 **Add your own recipes and tips here:**

DEODORIZER

Deodorizing Room Spray recipe # 1: 1 drop cinnamon oil, 3 drops of clove essential oil, 3 drops cedarwood essential oil, 6 drops tea tree essential oil, 7 drops of lemon essential oil. Mix in 2 cups water and use in a spray bottle.

Recipe # 2: You can make your natural home deodorizer and freshener by combining therapeutic scents like cinnamon, orange, lemon and cloves. And 2 drops of each to a spray bottle or diffuse.

Recipe # 3: Add 7 drops of cypress, 5 drops eucalyptus oil, 4 drops lemon, and 6 drops of pine to a 1 oz spray bottle with water for a disinfecting and revitalizing room spray.

Recipe # 4: Mix eucalyptus oil with lemon oil or tea tree oil for an anti-stink spray. Ideal for spraying bins.

Tip:
Add a few drops of eucalyptus oil to the vacuum and clothes dryer filters to freshen and sanitize.

Neroli: This essential oil can eliminate bad odors. It can be used on the body as a perfume or in rooms as room fresheners or vaporizers. This will not only drive away odor but will also disinfect the rooms against germs and toxins. Add a few drops to a spray bottle to banish odors and germs.

DISINFECTANT

Vinegar disinfectant:

1/2 cup white vinegar

6 drops of Lavender

Combine lavender oil to the spray bottle and fill with white vinegar. Shake to combine. Perfect for the bathroom and toilet. An alternative to chemical disinfectants and antibacterial sprays.

Basic disinfectant:

1 cup of rubbing alcohol

6 drops of lavender

6 drops of tea tree

6 drops of lemon

Clean spray bottle. Shake to combine. Perfect for disinfecting surfaces.

> ***Cypress room spray:*** *Add 6 drops cypress, 6 drops eucalyptus oil, 4 drops lemon oil, and 7 drops pine oil to a 1 oz spray bottle with water for a disinfecting and enlivening room spray.*

Lemon: Natural Disinfectant – Steer away from alcohol and bleach to disinfect your countertops and to clean a moldy shower. Add 35 drops lemon oil and 25 drops tea tree oil to 2 cups of water and add to a spray bottle (and a little bit of white vinegar) for a traditional cleaning favourite.

EAR INFECTION / EARACHE

Basil: Rubbing a combination of frankincense, coconut, and basil essential oil behind the ears and at the bottoms of your feet can speed up the time it takes to recover from ear infections while reducing pain and swelling. After rubbing into your feet, put on a pair of socks.

> ***Clove oil:*** *A mixture of warm clove oil and sesame oil is a good remedy for earaches.*

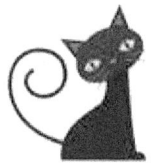 **Add your own recipes and tips here:**

EYE CARE

Clary sage: For eye care, add 2–3 drops of clary sage oil to a clean and warm washcloth; press cloth over closed eyes for 10 minutes.

> *Olive oil:* Use (high quality medical grade) castor oil eye drops to reduce symptoms of dry, red, itchy eyes, styes, conjunctivitis (Pink Eye), broken blood vessel in the eye, glaucoma and cataracts. Castor oil has strong anti-bacterial and anti-inflammatory properties.

Massage a small amount of the oil around the eyes to reduce wrinkles and dark circles. Also thickens eye lashes.

NOTE: NOT recommended for use with contacts in.

Apply no more than 2 drops into each eye before bed. Always make sure the eyes are clean, dry and without any makeup. For severe issues, apply the dosage again in the morning. Close your eyes and massage on and around the eye gently. If the eye area is too oily, dab area with a tissue to remove excess. Vision will be blurry, so treatment at night before bed is recommended.

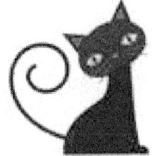 Add your own recipes and tips here:

HAIRCARE

Baking soda and apple cider vinegar: Before shampooing and conditioning, mix half a cup of each and wash through hair to remove bacteria, grease, and residue from hair naturally.

Basil: To strip away excess grease or build-up on your hair and promote shine, add a drop or two of basil oil to your shampoo.

Cedarwood essential oil can stimulate the hair follicles, increasing circulation to the scalp. Massage the oil into your scalp and let it sit for 30 minutes before rinsing. Add several drops to shampoo or conditioner bottles to add shine.

Eucalyptus oil: Before shampooing, add a few drops of eucalyptus oil with some coconut oil and massage into your scalp to give your hair a nice moisturizing pick-me-up. Cover head with shower cap and leave for half an hour. This is especially great to fight dandruff and an itchy scalp. Also, eucalyptus is used as a natural remedy for lice in replacement of chemical treatments.

Lavender essential oil is useful for hair care as it has proven to be very effective on lice, lice eggs, and nits. Furthermore, lavender essential oil has also been shown to be very helpful in the treatment of hair loss, particularly for patients who suffer from alopecia

Rosemary: Mix 25 drops of rosemary oil in a cup of water and then rub the mixture onto your scalp and on your hair strands. This is believed to be able to slow graying, stop dandruff, increase growth, and keep the scalp free of irritation or infection.

> **Rosemary:** *Hair Thickener – Put 5 drops of rosemary oil on scalp and massage in after showers.*

Homemade Conditioner

This homemade conditioner helps to restore the hair's natural pH, thus rehydrating the hair. The result is soft, luscious and healthy hair.

Total Time: 2 minutes. Uses: 20–30

INGREDIENTS:

1 cup water

2 tablespoons apple cider vinegar

10 drops of geranium oil

BPA-free plastic bottles or glass bottle with dispenser.

How to customize your conditioner:

Rosemary or sage essential oils for all types of hair.

Lemon, bergamot or tea tree essential oils are ideal for oily hair.

Lavender, sandalwood or geranium essential oils for dry hair or dandruff.

DIRECTIONS:

Mix ingredients together in 1 cup of water. Add to spray bottle.

Shake bottle before using and then spray hair.

Leave in hair for five minutes, then rinse.

Geranium: Mix 5-7 drops with ½ fl. Oz. of Olive Old to create a luscious hair oil treatment to breathe new life into dull and limp hair! This sweet smelling essential oil contains antioxidants that reinvigorate limp damaged hair.

Grapefruit. Add a few drops of grapefruit essential oil to your shampoo or conditioner to reduce the build up of grease, sweat, and bacteria while adding volume and shine to your hair.

Add your own recipes and tips here:

HEADACHES

Rosemary for a headache. Rub your temples with a little rosemary essential oil. Rosemary is a stimulating oil which increases circulation under the skin, relieving pain & muscle tension. Rosemary oil releases tension and calms anxiety, which may have been the cause of the headache.

Blend: Add 2 drops of rosemary essential oil to a teaspoon of carrier oil. I like to use coconut oil. Massage the mix onto your temples. This blend can also be used on joint pain. Adding 1 drop of peppermint oil may also help.

Sprinkle rosemary oil on a tissue in inhale for headache relief, or add to a water bottle for a spritz. Diffusing is also ideal. You may also like to add a couple of drops of rosemary and lavender to your pillow when you rest. Adding a few drops to your warm bath water is also very relaxing after a long day.

Cinnamon: Because the active compounds in cinnamon oil helps increase circulation by expanding blood vessels, headache pain can be reduced by diffusing 4 drops of cinnamon essential oil.

Add your own recipes and tips here:

HOUSEHOLD CLEANERS

Note before you start:

Never blend essential oils in metal or plastic contains or bottles. Some oils may create a chemical reaction. When it comes to mixing or storing essential oils, it's always best to use glass.

Eucalyptus Cleaner:

15 drops of eucalyptus oil.

1/2 cup white vinegar water.

Add the eucalyptus oil and the vinegar in a spray bottle and fill with water and shake. Ideal for cleaning bathtubs, showers, bench-tops, and hand basins.

> **Lemon:** *Goo-Be-Gone – Un-stick the sticky goo your kids leave behind with stickers and gum with lemon oil. Do a patch test on some surfaces before using.*

Lime: is excellent at removing sticker residue and gum from surfaces.

Orange Cleaner:

15 drops of Orange Oil

3 tablespoons bicarbonate of soda

Add all ingredients to spray bottle and add water - shake well. An excellent combination to replace chemical cleaners in the kitchen.

Peppermint Cleaner:

10 peppermint

5 rosemary

5 lemon

5 eucalyptus

5 lavender

Add all ingredients to spray bottle and add water - shake well. Perfect for cleaning out kitchen bins.

Glass cleaner:

Chemicals in cleaning supplies can be hazardous to your health and the environment.

What You Need:

500ml Spray Bottle – glass.

1 1/2 cup white vinegar

1/2 cup distilled water

4 drops of Lemon or Lime, and 4 drops of Wild Orange.

Directions:

Add vinegar, water, and essential oils to spray bottle and shake before using.

Homemade Melaleuca (tea tree) and Lemon Household Cleaner.

Most commercial cleaners are made with synthetic fragrances and harmful chemicals. This Homemade Household Cleaner is just as effective due to tea tree's antimicrobial properties. Made with only 4 ingredients, it's easy and fast to make.

Total Time: 2 minutes. Serves: 30-90INGREDIENTS:

1 cup water

½ cup distilled white vinegar

15 drops tea tree oil

15 drops lemon

Glass Spray bottle

DIRECTIONS:

Fill spray bottle with ingredients. Shake before each use.

LAUNDRY SOAP

Avoid toxic chemicals found in most store-bought products and make your own antibacterial, deodorizing, laundry soap.

Takes about 5 minutes.

14 loads of washing depending on your load size. Approximately half a cup per average load. Use more for heavily soiled items.

INGREDIENTS:

2 bars Castile soap bar – grated.

2 and ½ cups Borax

2 and ½ cups washing soda

1 and ½ cups baking soda

8 drops basil essential oil

8 drops of lemon essential oil

10 drops of lavender essential oil

12 drops of peppermint essential oil

DIRECTIONS:

Combine all ingredients and store in an air-tight container.

MENOPAUSE

Menopause isn't a disease but rather a natural period of change in a woman's life. It can start occurring as early as the mid-thirties, although this is not common. For most women menopause usually creeps in around their 40's. You might wake up with the occasional night sweats, or you start getting headaches more frequently or feeling irritable. The average age for the onset of menopause is usually fifty-one. Some women experience only minor symptoms, while others experience quite severe symptoms. For some women, it can last just two or three years, but on average, symptoms can last up to seven years. Seven. Long. Years... That's a long time to feel miserable.

Many essential oils mimic estrogen in the body, tricking it into believing that it's still getting the estrogen, and offering many women relief from the symptoms of menopause.

Night sweats:
Of all of the essential oils, peppermint really tops on the list. The menthol in peppermint oil makes your brain think that whatever part of your body you apply it to is cooler. Your skin will absorb the oil and distribute this "cooling" effect over the body. Never apply peppermint oil directly to the face. If you want to use it on your face, you'll need to dilute about 4 drops of peppermint oil in one tablespoon of carrier oil such as jojoba oil or coconut oil.

Other essential oils that may help you are lime, lemon, orange, grapefruit, clary sage, geranium, and cypress. Try making a spritz by putting about 20 drops of your favorite oil in a spray bottle and mix it with 1 cup of water. Mist away for instant cooling relief that will last for hours. Diffusing essential oils in your home and workplace will also offer you some comfort, especially at night.

Do you feel like Dr Jekyll and Mr Hyde?

Feeling irritable with everyone around you or want to cry at the drop of a hat? One of my friends even went as far as wanting to throw herself under a bus, while another flew into uncharacteristic rages at any who crossed her path at the drop of a hat. The female version of Dr Jekyll and Mr Hyde, I kid you not. Most women find that having a bath filled with essential oils can help regulate their emotions. Some of the best oils for a relaxing soak are lavender, ylang-ylang, Roman chamomile, sandalwood, and valerian. Add about 20 to 40 drops to your bathwater for instant relief. Again, using a diffuser will also offer much-needed relief. Depending on which scent you like the best, you might choose to keep a small bottle in your purse to dab on a tissue an inhale when you feel you are about to lose it.

Lavender: Having problems with your mood swings during menopause is completely natural. However, in order to spare yourself from the issues which derive from this, you can diffuse a few drops of lavender to induce a feeling of calmness and relaxation.

For pain relief, try sweet marjoram, rosemary, thyme, eucalyptus, German or Roman chamomile, lavender, and peppermint. Chamomile, sweet marjoram, and lavender will leave you feeling more relaxed, so these are ideal for night time use. You can mix your favorite essential oils with some almond oil or coconut oil and massage into the skin for almost instant relief.

Herbal teas can also offer some relief.

Lubrication.

One of the most frustrating symptoms of menopause is vaginal dryness, making sex very uncomfortable. Try mixing clary sage, 1 or 2 drops, with a tablespoon of good quality carrier oil such as coconut oil or olive oil. Apply at least once per day.

Fatigued?

Menopause can come with episodes of fatigue. Sometimes a catnap can go a long way to making you feel more energized. When you can't find the time to grab a snooze in your busy schedule, try some basil, rosemary, black pepper, ginger, eucalyptus, and nutmeg or peppermint essential oils in a room diffuser or a spray bottle. Prevention is always better than the cure. Before you begin to feel rundown, turn the diffuser on or fill up your spritzer bottle. Stay hydrated. Make up a jug of herbal tea, let it cool then put it in the fridge. Add ice cubes, sprigs of rosemary, ginger, cucumber for a refreshing pick-me-up.

Insomnia.

The thing with menopause is that you can feel so washed out and tired during the day, but when it's time to go to bed, you can't sleep. Or if you do manage to fall asleep, you wake up after just a few hours and can't get back to sleep. This is when using a room diffuser really comes in handy.

The best oils for insomnia are

Lavender

Roman or German chamomile

Valerian

Clary sage

Sweet marjoram.

> *Put a few drops into your diffuser before going to bed or sprinkle a few drops on your pillow.*

The most common way to use essential oils are to either mixed in a suitable quality oil carrier and apply directly to the skin, add to a warm bath, or in your room diffuser.

Again, using a spray bottle filled with water and peppermint oil for instant relief from hot flashes works wonders. Get creative. Experiment with different oils until you find ones that work best for you.

Avoid the known triggers:
- Stress
- Excessive use of caffeine – opt for herbal teas instead
- Heat
- Sugar
- Alcohol
- Smoking
- Certain medications (speak with your health practitioner)

Frankincense essential oil is also known for regulating the production of oestrogen in women. Therefore, it could reduce the risk of cyst formation in your uterus as well as other serious conditions. It's also known for regulating the menstrual cycle of women who are in their premenopausal age.

Jasmine oil - Either as an aromatherapy treatment or applying it directly to the skin can help decrease emotional and physical symptoms of menopause and work as a natural remedy for menopause relief.

Oregano - This oil is beneficial in regulating menstruation and delaying the onset of menopause. Those suffering from obstructed menses may also find relief by using oregano essential oil. As an emmenagogue, it can help a woman reduce her symptoms of oncoming menopause, including mood imbalance and hormonal shifts.

Always remember that you are not alone during this time.

Add your own recipes and tips here:

MOLD AND MILDEW

Blend:

2 cups of water

2 teaspoons of tea tree oil

8 drops of basil

Add to a clean spray bottle – shake.

Ideal for bathroom and kitchen surfaces.

Eucalyptus oil is great for killing mold in your home. In a spray bottle, mix eucalyptus with other oils such as clove and tea tree oil to cleanse the air and uphold a mold-free home.

> *Tea tree: Spray tea tree oil cleaner onto shower curtains, your laundry machine, dishwasher or toilet to kill mold.*

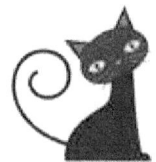 **Add your own recipes and tips here:**

NAIL CARE

Lemongrass: Combine lemongrass oil with Melaleuca in order to create a DIY nail-polish. This can attribute for healthy nails and toenails.

Add your own recipes and tips here:

NAUSEA

Clove oil is helpful in reducing nausea and vomiting. Diffuse or apply a few drops to pillows at night for positive effects.

Add your own recipes and tips here:

ORAL

Basil: To remove bacteria and odour from your mouth, add 5 drops of basil oil and 5 drops of peppermint to a tablespoon of coconut oil and swish around your mouth for 2 minutes. This also helps protect your teeth and gums from toothaches, ulcers, sores and viral blisters.

Bergamot: Add a few drops of bergamot oil to a glass of water to make a mouthwash or gargle preparation or add a 2 - 3 drops to your toothpaste and brush as normal.

Cardamom: Add 5 drops of cardamom to water and gargle. Cardamom disinfects and eliminates bad breath.

Cilantro/coriander: It reduces bad breath and eliminates mouth and body odor when used either internally or externally. When consumed or ingested, the typical aroma of coriander oil mixes with sweat and fights body odor as well as oral. Cilantro also helps to inhibit bacterial growth in your mouth and around your sweat glands, thereby fighting the odour. Add a few drops to water, swirl around your mouth and expel.

Clove: Before bed, gargle four ounces of water with one drop of clove oil. You can also add a single drop to your toothpaste before brushing your teeth.

Cumin: For an antiseptic mouth rinse, add one drop to half a glass of water and gargle.

Eucalyptus oil reduces cavities, plaque, and gum disease. Add a few drops with half a glass of water for a natural mouthwash and gargle.

Fennel: Place one drop of fennel essential oil on your toothbrush when brushing to provide antimicrobial benefits for the gums.

Frankincense: Many people use frankincense to relieve oral health problems naturally. The antiseptic qualities of this oil can help prevent gingivitis, bad breath, cavities, toothaches, mouth sores and other infections from occurring. Add a couple of drops to water for mouthwash before brushing your teeth.

> ***Lemon:*** *Teeth Whitener – Mix a few drops of lemon essential oil, baking soda, and coconut oil and rub on your teeth for 2 minutes and then rinse.*

Tea tree: Mix tea tree oil with coconut oil and baking soda for an amazing homemade toothpaste.

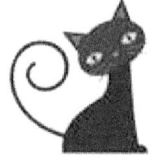 **Add your own recipes and tips here:**

PERFUME

Homemade Jasmine Oil Perfume

Ingredients:

30 drops jasmine oil

5 drops vanilla essential oil

5 drops lavender essential oil

5 drops orange essential oil

2 tablespoons vodka

1 tablespoon orange blossom water (or distilled water)

Directions:

Mix the essential oil blend with the vodka in a glass mason jar or bottle and leave it to sit on a countertop for two days. Keep it covered and somewhere that's room temperature and away from the sun.

Add the orange blossom water or distilled water and stir together. Add the mixture to a glass bottle. Keep the mix somewhere around room temperature, and use on your skin, clothes, sheets, rugs, etc.

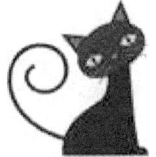 Add your own recipes and tips here:

PICK-ME-UP

Rosemary for remembrance. Rosemary essential oil is an excellent brain and nerve tonic. Inhaling rosemary essential is often used by students during exams because it increases concentration. It stimulates mental activity and is an ideal good remedy for depression, mental fatigue, and forgetfulness. Inhaling the fragrance rosemary oil also lifts your spirits immediately. Whenever you are tired, try inhaling a little rosemary oil to renew your mental energy.

Blend: Add a couple of drops to a carrier oil and massage into your temples. Also, a good treatment for headaches. Add a few drops to water and make a refreshing spritz. Leave the bottle in the fridge on a hot day for an extra boost. If studying in your home, try diffusing 6 drops of oil into a diffuser. Add a couple of drops of peppermint and orange oil to boost a tired brain.

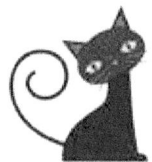 Add your own recipes and tips here:

SKINCARE

Basil. Acne is caused by the build-up of bacteria and excess oil. Basil oil is an ideal home remedy for this problem. Using a clean cotton ball, apply 1 - 2 drops of basil oil with coconut oil to the affected area morning and night.

Cedarwood. Make your own face scrub by combining 6 drops of cedarwood essential oil with enough Epsom salt and coconut oil to make a paste to cover your face. Mix these ingredients until you get a rough and slightly oily texture — then use the mixture to exfoliate your face and help eliminate acne.

Clary sage: Create a mix of clary sage oil and a carrier oil (like coconut or jojoba) at a 1:1 ratio. Apply the mixture directly to your face, neck, and body.

Helichrysum Skin Rejuvenation blend: 12 drops helichrysum essential oil, 6 drops carrot seed essential oil, 6 drops rosemary oil in 15 ml rosehip oil, and 1 teaspoon of coconut oil.

Helichrysum: Prevents hives, redness, blemishes, rashes and shaving irritation. If you have a rash or poison ivy, applying helichrysum mixed with lavender oil can help calm and soothe any itching.

Apply 2-4 drops of undiluted oil directly on the skin to the affected area or desired location.

Or – 2 – 4 drops on sore bodies to soothe, just add it to your favorite massage oil and rub.

Lemon: Face mask – Lemon essential oil uses for skin can improve your complexion and leave your skin soft and supple. Mix lemon oil with baking soda and honey for a natural face mask. Leave for half an hour then wash off with warm water.

Melissa: To treat skin conditions, such as eczema, use five drops per ounce of carrier oil, primarily for use on the face. Alternatively, you can add five drops to a moisturizer or a spray bottle with water and spritz it on your face.

> *Melissa: To treats cold sores and herpes, apply 2 to 3 diluted drops of melissa topically to the area of concern.*

Honey Face Wash

Total Time: 2 minutes. Serves: 30

INGREDIENTS:

1 tablespoon coconut oil

3 tablespoons honey

1 tablespoon apple cider vinegar

20 drops helichrysum essential oil

2 capsules of live probiotics

DIRECTIONS:

Mix all ingredients together and blend with a hand blender. Pour into a jar and store in cool place.

Add your own recipes and tips here:

SUNBURN

Sunburn Soother Recipe 1

Ingredients:

1/8 cup of coconut oil.

1/8 teaspoon of vitamin E oil.

A few drops of lavender oil.

Small bowl and spoon.

Small jar with a twist cap.

Directions

Place the coconut oil in the bowl.

Blend the oil. It may be solid at first, so you will need to smooth out any lumps.

Add the vitamin E oil.

Mix thoroughly. You'll find the oil easier to stir at this point.

Add in the drops of lavender oil.

Mix thoroughly.

Spoon the oil into a small jar or container with a twist lid.

Store the jar away from heat or sunlight.

To use your coconut oil sunburn remedy, merely place some oil on your fingertips and rub it into the sunburn. Massage it in until your skin absorbs it. Leave it to dry for a few minutes.

> *You can use this remedy on most areas of your body. Avoid the areas around your eyes, or placing directly in your ears.*

Sunburn Soother Recipe 2

Total Time: 20-30 minutes.

INGREDIENTS:

12 drops frankincense essential oil

10 drops helichrysum essential oil

3/4 cup coconut oil

2 tablespoons shea butter

Glass jar

DIRECTIONS:

Combine all ingredients in a jar.

Place a saucepan with two inches of water on the stove over medium to low heat.

Place the jar in the saucepan and stir contents until ingredients begin to melt. Once all ingredients are combined, store in a cool place for later use.

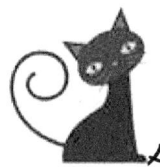Add your own recipes and tips here:

HEAD LICE

Tea tree oil has natural antimicrobial, antibacterial and anti-inflammatory properties. Combination of tea tree oil along with lavender oil kills lice eggs. It is advisable to do a skin test first whenever applying essential oils to your skin.

Prepare a solution of shampoo and tea tree oil – tea tree oil by itself may cause skin irritations, so it is advisable to mix with a few drops of shampoo before using. For best results, add a few drops of lavender or coconut oil. Coconut oil will help by suffocating the lice. Mix your solution well to blend.

Apply the mixture to the hair. Make sure you apply the mixture directly to the scalp. Once applied, cover your head with a shower cap and leave it for around 20-30 minutes. If you experience any itchiness or burning, wash out – you may be experiencing an allergic reaction.

Massage mixture into your scalp while rinsing your hair with warm water.

Apply hair conditioner then rinse once again.

Use a lice comb to comb through the hair. Starting at the scalp, comb through to the ends. If you have longer hair, separate hair into smaller sections to make combing easier. Be thorough. For best results, repeat this process regularly for 2-3 weeks.

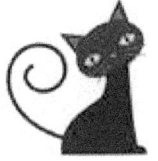 Add your own recipes and tips here:

PARASITES

People who eat uncooked meat, especially pork are most likely to have parasites because the parasite's eggs are not destroyed during the cooking process.

Parasites love sugar. The best way to starve the parasites is through using healthy fasting and cleansing strategies while eliminating as much sugar and grains as possible from the diet.

The most common types of internal parasites that affect humans include:

Tapeworms

Pinworms

Roundworms

Hookworms

Always consult your doctor before ingesting essential oils. Ingest only 100% pure certified organic food grade essential oils.

The following is a list of things to avoid:

Alcohol

Caffeine

Fermented foods

Gluten-containing grains

Milk and dairy products

Sugar

Parasites usually cause dysentery, diarrhea, vomiting, stomach pain, constipation, feeling hungry all the time, or a loss of appetite.

A parasite infestation can cause severe health problems, especially if the larvae get into other parts of the body from the gut.

> ***Oregano oil***: *Add 2 drops of food grade wild oil of oregano to water and drink. Because the taste is quite overpowering, you may prefer to add the oil to a capsule. Take one two times a day **for 3 days.***

Alternatively, use 2 drops of oregano oil in water with freshly squeezed lemon and drink this three times a day. Clove works just as well so you could also substitute or use clove oil with oregano oil. Ginger, wormwood, and black walnut are also commonly used in anti-parasitic strategies.

Castor Oil Pack

What you need

1 tbsp. castor oil

5 drops clove

3 drops oregano

3 drops thyme

Hot water bottle

Method.

Mix the essential oils in the castor oil until well combined. Rub it deeply onto your belly in a clockwise motion, from the belly button going outwards. Place a hot water bottle on top to create heat for 30 minutes.

Notes:

PETS

Warning: Do not keep pets in an enclosed, poorly ventilated area while using essential oils. Unlike dogs, people, and horses, cats lack a liver enzyme (glucuronyl tranferase) required to break down the components of most essential oils.

Though there are essential oils that are toxic to pets, there are a few essential oils that can be used to help them. Essential oils can be quite safe for our dogs and cats and even very useful, but only when the correct amount is diluted well and used correctly. Always check before using undiluted essential oil on yourself or your pet.

Note about Animal Use: Certain oils can be very toxic to cats, dogs, and birds, especially if they are not therapeutic quality. Pine and citrus products and oils, in particular, should not be used. Please consult your vet if you have any questions about applying essential oil to your pet. If you pet shows signs of salivation, vomiting, diarrhea, depression, weakness, consult your veterinarian straight away.

Here are the top 5 list essential oils for cats that are very safe.
Cedarwood Essential Oil
Frankincense Essential Oil
Geranium Essential Oil
Helichrysum Essential Oil
Lavender Essential Oil

How do I use Essential Oils with Cats?
Essential oils for cats should be highly diluted with a high-grade pure vegetable oil. Dilute essential oils for cats (and all other smaller animals) at least 50:1 (fifty drops of dilution oil to one drop of essential oil).

Those are just a few of the essential oils you can use on your pets – with caution. If you are interested in learning more information, you can talk to a holistic veterinarian for more suggestions.

The use of essential oils on cats is typically discouraged. In certain circumstances, some oils can be used to treat specific ailments under a veterinarian's supervision when diluted, otherwise, they should be avoided.

You can find out more about essential oils for pets by downloading the FREE ebook > http://amzn.to/2BLc7ZN

Or buy the print book > http://amzn.to/2AxgabY

Add your own recipes and tips here:

HERBAL REMEDIES FOR ADD

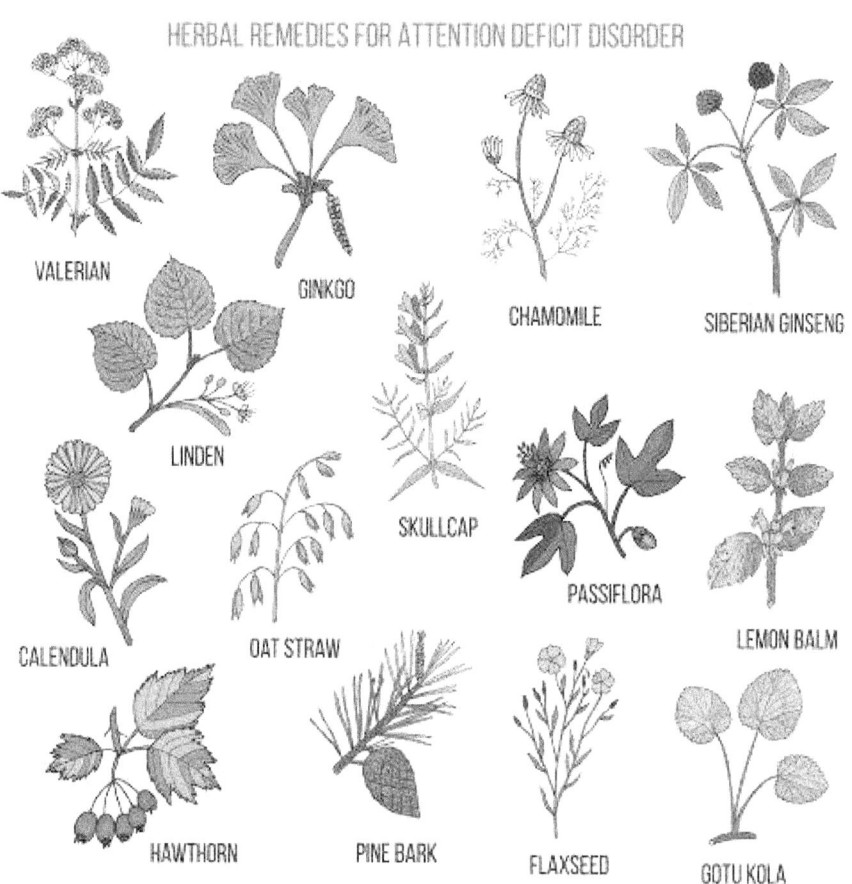

HERBAL REMEDIES FOR ATTENTION DEFICIT DISORDER

VALERIAN

GINKGO

CHAMOMILE

SIBERIAN GINSENG

LINDEN

SKULLCAP

PASSIFLORA

LEMON BALM

CALENDULA

OAT STRAW

HAWTHORN

PINE BARK

FLAXSEED

GOTU KOLA

ANTI-AGING HERBS

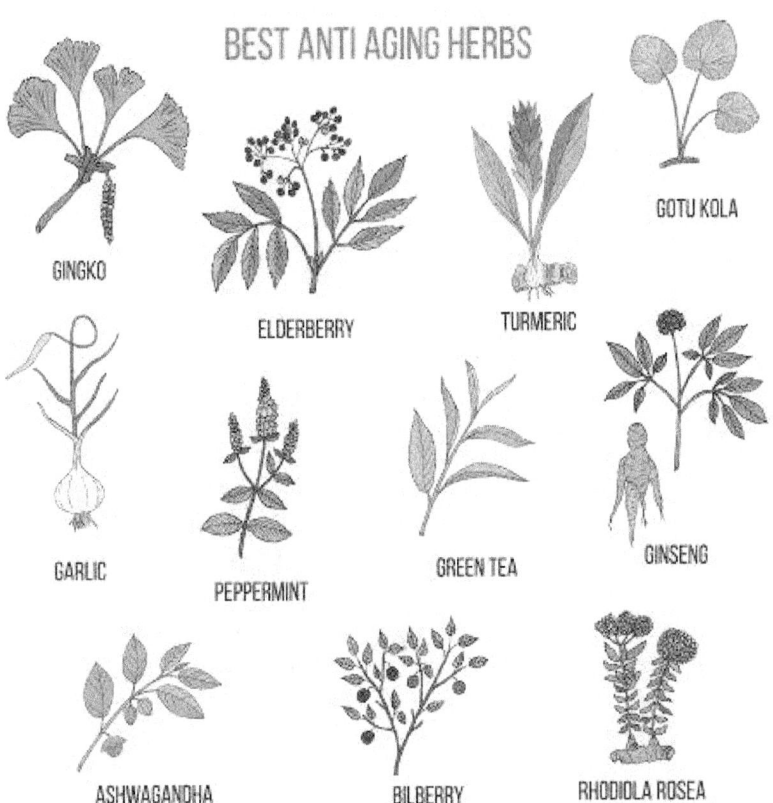

BEST ANTI AGING HERBS

GINGKO

ELDERBERRY

TURMERIC

GOTU KOLA

GARLIC

PEPPERMINT

GREEN TEA

GINSENG

ASHWAGANDHA

BILBERRY

RHODIOLA ROSEA

ANTI-INFLAMMATORY HERBS

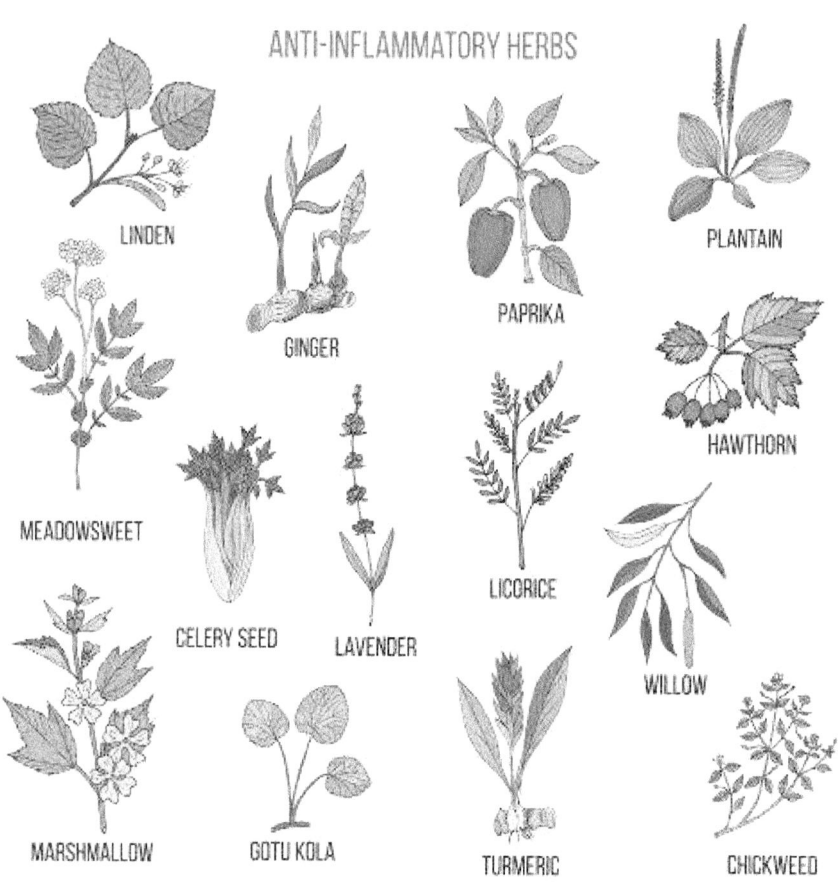

ANTIMICROBIAL HERBS

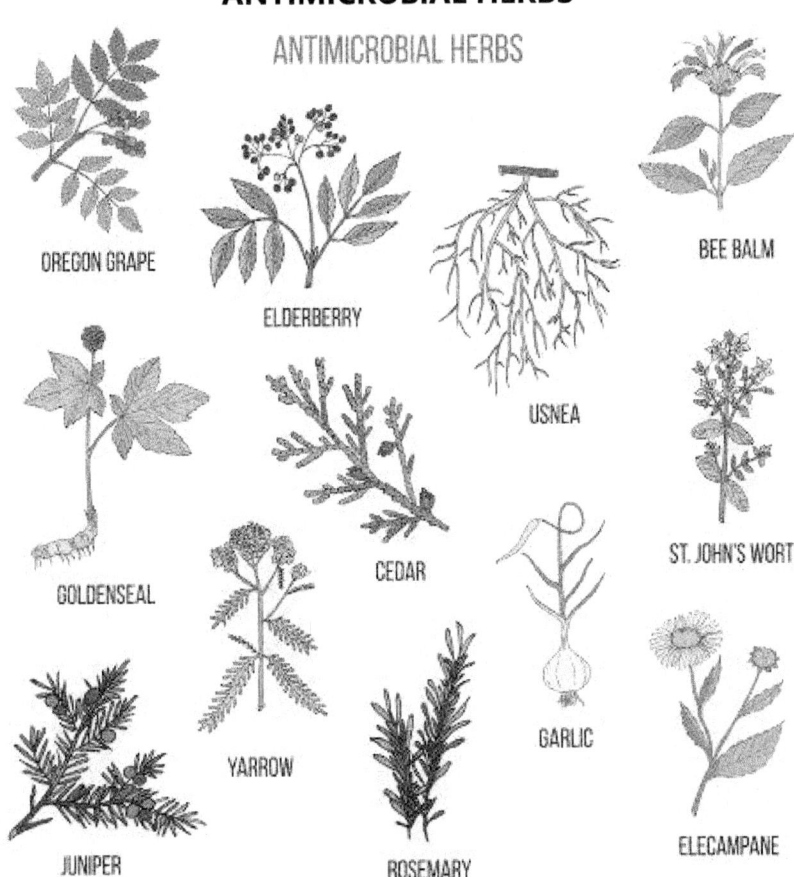

ANTIMICROBIAL HERBS

OREGON GRAPE

ELDERBERRY

USNEA

BEE BALM

GOLDENSEAL

CEDAR

ST. JOHN'S WORT

YARROW

GARLIC

JUNIPER

ROSEMARY

ELECAMPANE

COMMON COLD

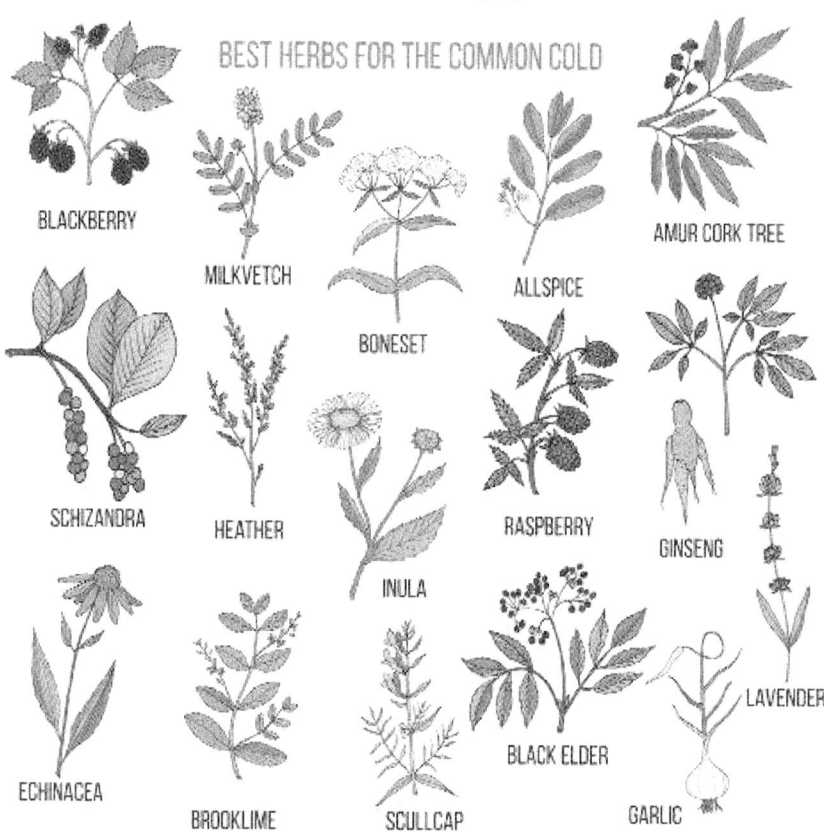

BEST HERBS FOR THE COMMON COLD

BLACKBERRY

MILKVETCH

BONESET

ALLSPICE

AMUR CORK TREE

SCHIZANDRA

HEATHER

INULA

RASPBERRY

GINSENG

ECHINACEA

BROOKLIME

SCULLCAP

BLACK ELDER

GARLIC

LAVENDER

DEPRESSION

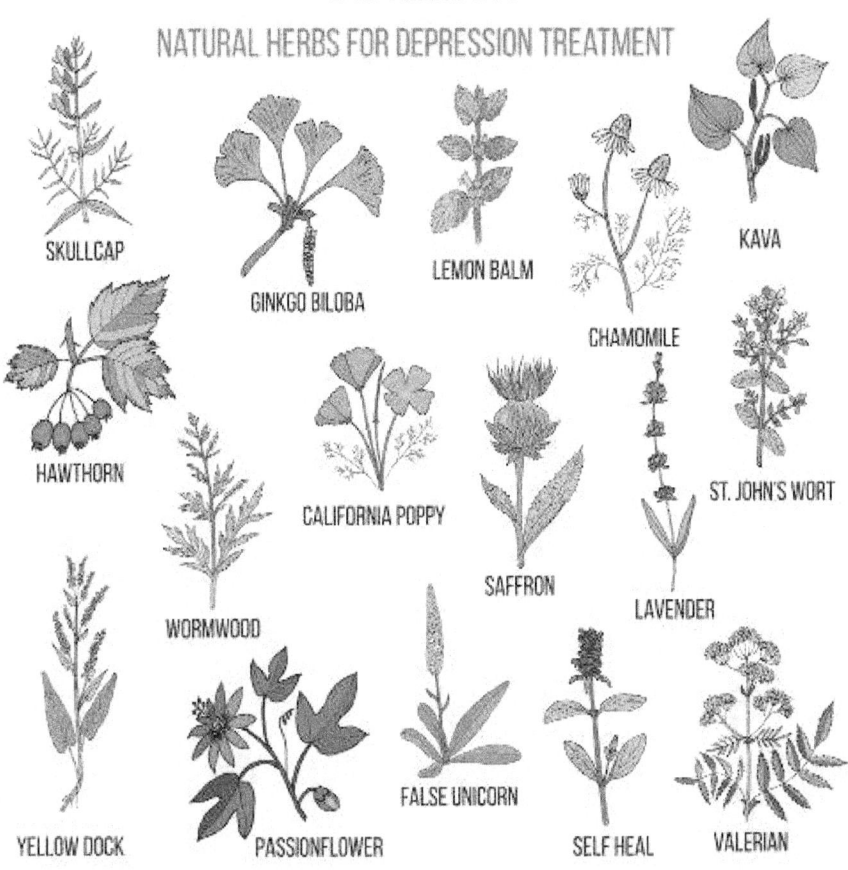

NATURAL HERBS FOR DEPRESSION TREATMENT

SKULLCAP

GINKGO BILOBA

LEMON BALM

CHAMOMILE

KAVA

HAWTHORN

CALIFORNIA POPPY

SAFFRON

ST. JOHN'S WORT

LAVENDER

WORMWOOD

YELLOW DOCK

PASSIONFLOWER

FALSE UNICORN

SELF HEAL

VALERIAN

FLU

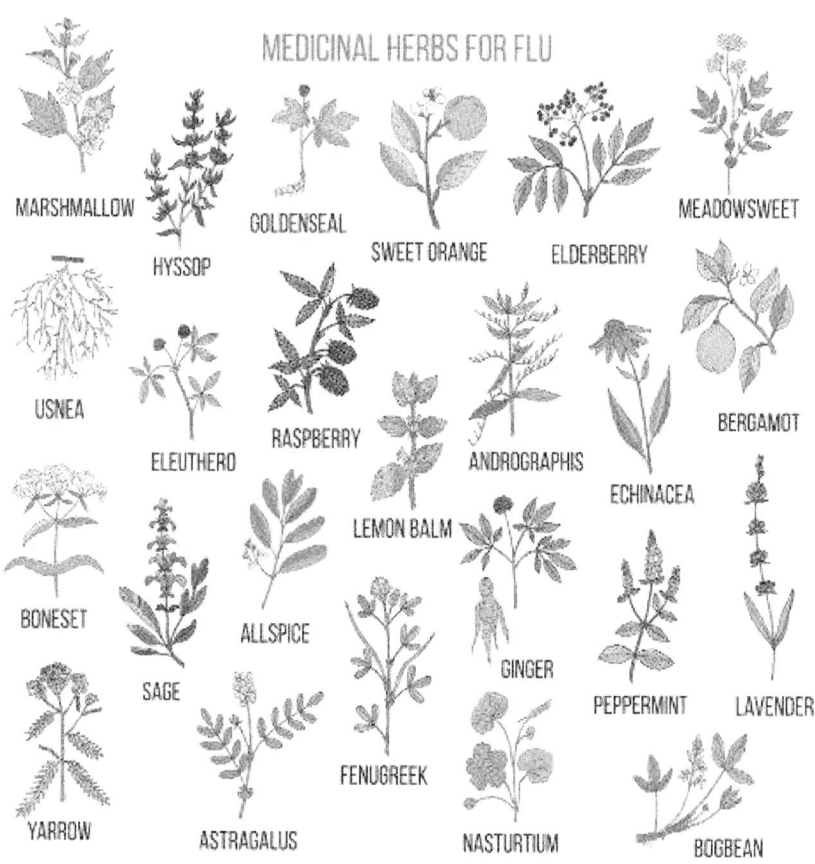

MEDICINAL HERBS FOR FLU

MARSHMALLOW

HYSSOP

GOLDENSEAL

SWEET ORANGE

ELDERBERRY

MEADOWSWEET

USNEA

ELEUTHERO

RASPBERRY

LEMON BALM

ANDROGRAPHIS

ECHINACEA

BERGAMOT

BONESET

SAGE

ALLSPICE

GINGER

PEPPERMINT

LAVENDER

YARROW

ASTRAGALUS

FENUGREEK

NASTURTIUM

BOGBEAN

HAIR GROWTH

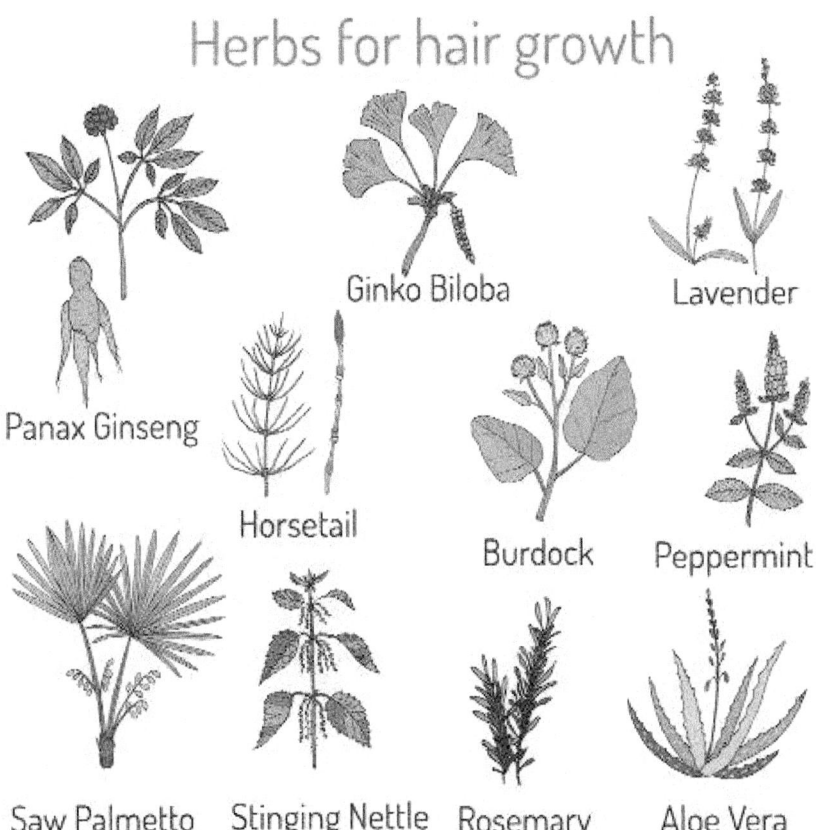

Herbs for hair growth

Panax Ginseng

Ginko Biloba

Lavender

Horsetail

Burdock

Peppermint

Saw Palmetto

Stinging Nettle

Rosemary

Aloe Vera

HEARTBURN

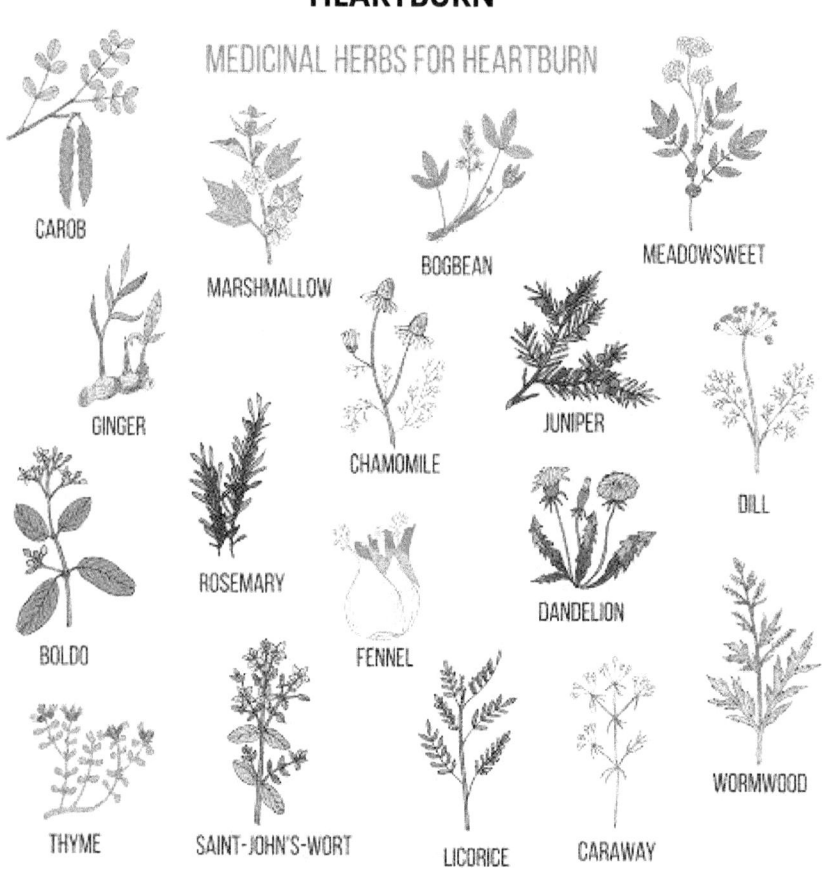

MEDICINAL HERBS FOR HEARTBURN

CAROB

MARSHMALLOW

BOGBEAN

MEADOWSWEET

GINGER

CHAMOMILE

JUNIPER

DILL

BOLDO

ROSEMARY

FENNEL

DANDELION

WORMWOOD

THYME

SAINT-JOHN'S-WORT

LICORICE

CARAWAY

IRRITABLE BOWEL SYNDROME

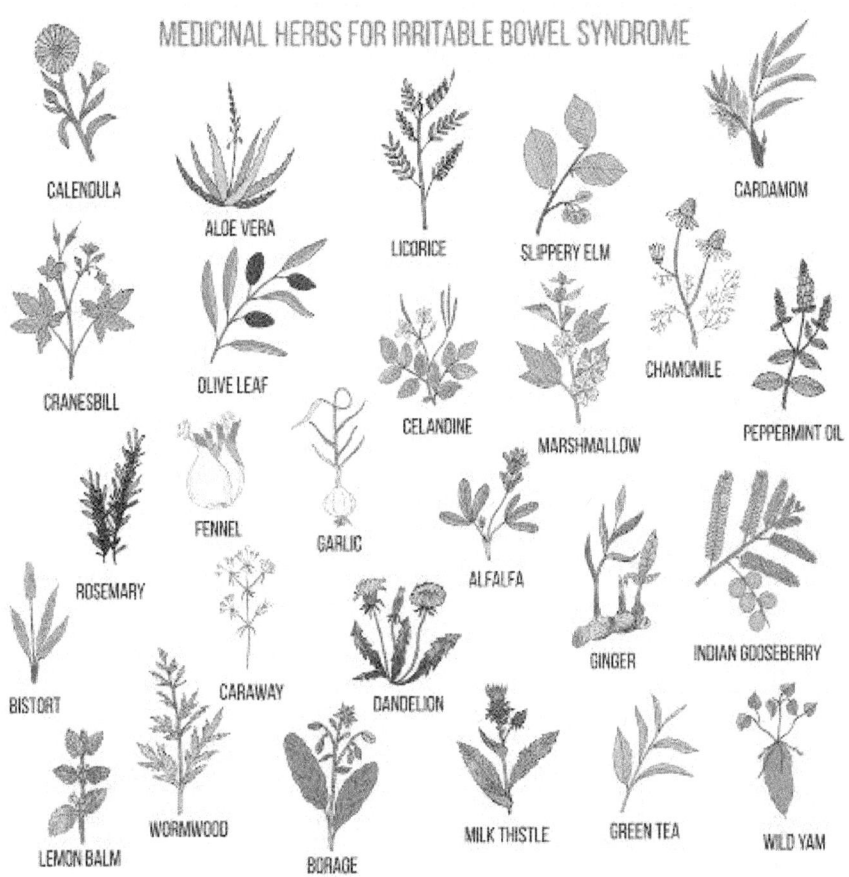

MEDICINAL HERBS FOR IRRITABLE BOWEL SYNDROME

CALENDULA

ALOE VERA

LICORICE

SLIPPERY ELM

CARDAMOM

CRANESBILL

OLIVE LEAF

CELANDINE

MARSHMALLOW

CHAMOMILE

PEPPERMINT OIL

ROSEMARY

FENNEL

GARLIC

ALFALFA

GINGER

INDIAN GOOSEBERRY

BISTORT

CARAWAY

DANDELION

MILK THISTLE

GREEN TEA

WILD YAM

LEMON BALM

WORMWOOD

BORAGE

IMMUNE SYSTEM

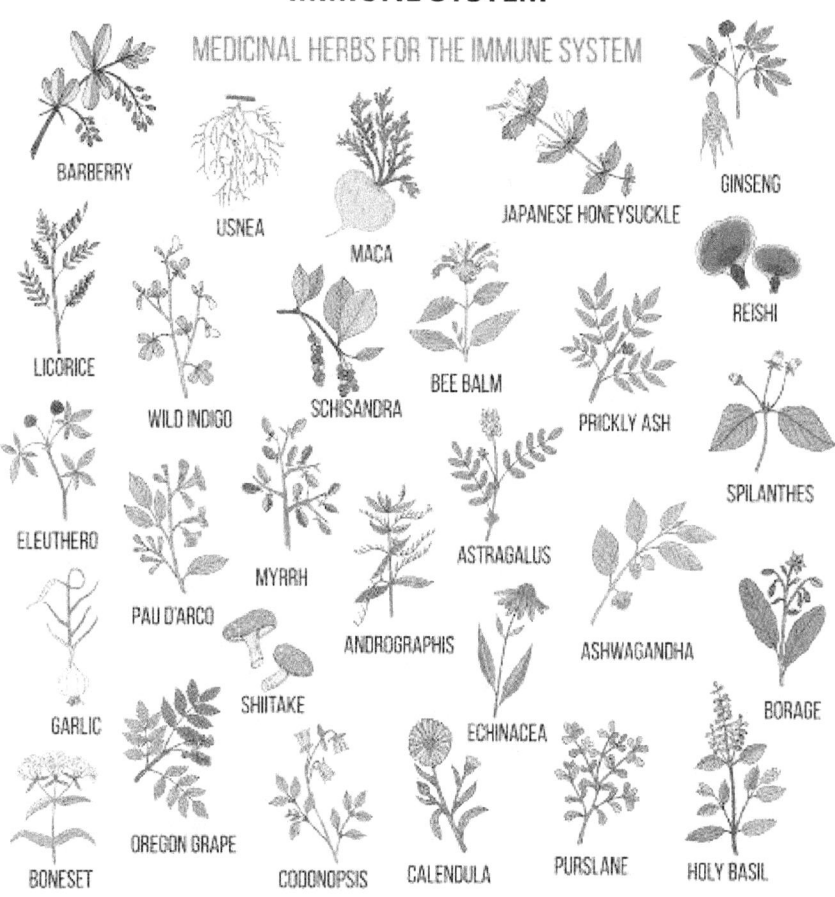

MEDICINAL HERBS FOR THE IMMUNE SYSTEM

BARBERRY

USNEA

MACA

JAPANESE HONEYSUCKLE

GINSENG

REISHI

LICORICE

WILD INDIGO

SCHISANDRA

BEE BALM

PRICKLY ASH

SPILANTHES

ELEUTHERO

MYRRH

ASTRAGALUS

PAU D'ARCO

ANDROGRAPHIS

ASHWAGANDHA

BORAGE

GARLIC

SHIITAKE

ECHINACEA

OREGON GRAPE

BONESET

CODONOPSIS

CALENDULA

PURSLANE

HOLY BASIL

PAIN RELIEF

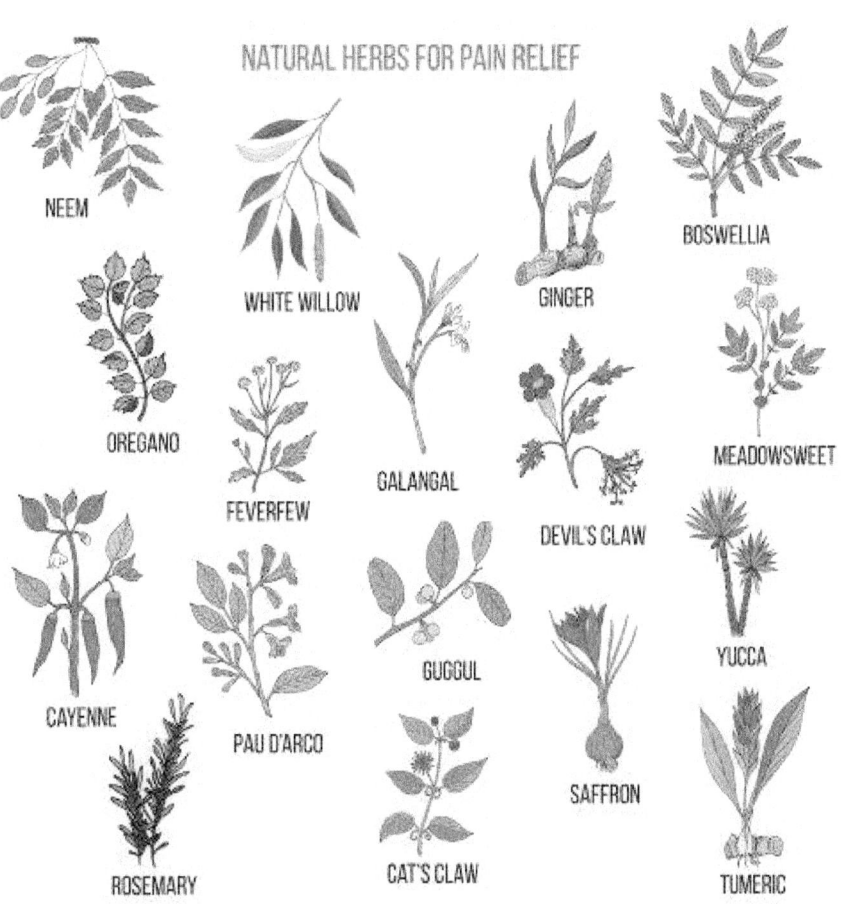

NATURAL HERBS FOR PAIN RELIEF

NEEM

WHITE WILLOW

GINGER

BOSWELLIA

OREGANO

FEVERFEW

GALANGAL

DEVIL'S CLAW

MEADOWSWEET

CAYENNE

PAU D'ARCO

GUGGUL

YUCCA

SAFFRON

ROSEMARY

CAT'S CLAW

TUMERIC

PSORIASIS

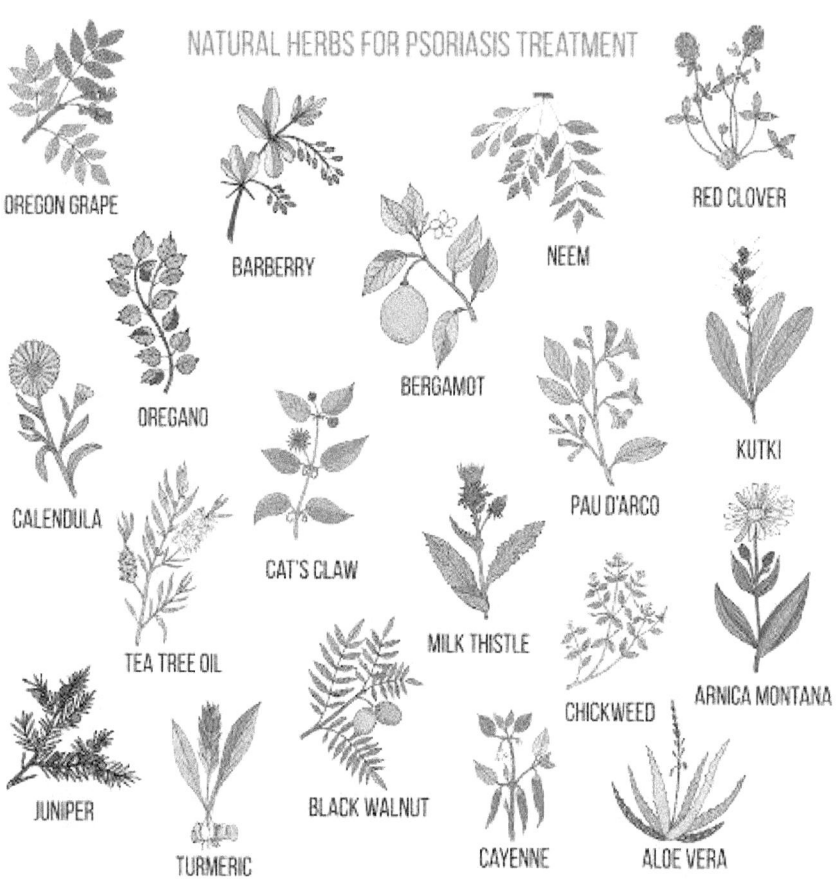

NATURAL HERBS FOR PSORIASIS TREATMENT

OREGON GRAPE

BARBERRY

NEEM

RED CLOVER

OREGANO

BERGAMOT

KUTKI

CALENDULA

CAT'S CLAW

PAU D'ARCO

TEA TREE OIL

MILK THISTLE

ARNICA MONTANA

CHICKWEED

JUNIPER

BLACK WALNUT

TURMERIC

CAYENNE

ALOE VERA

SLEEP AND RELAXATION

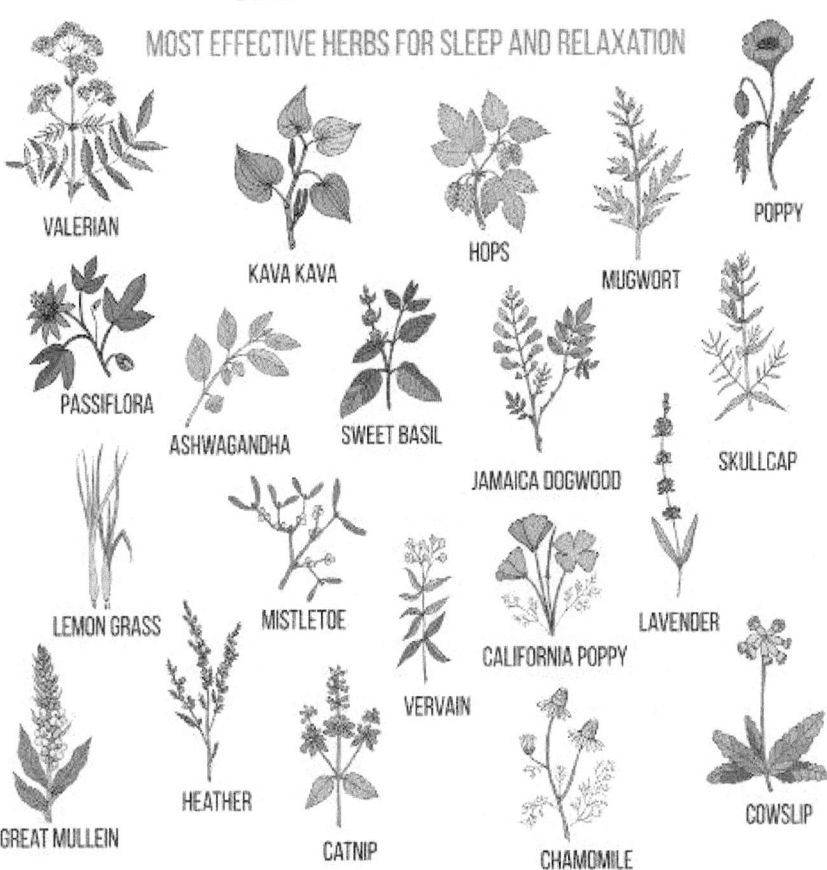

MOST EFFECTIVE HERBS FOR SLEEP AND RELAXATION

VALERIAN

KAVA KAVA

HOPS

MUGWORT

POPPY

PASSIFLORA

ASHWAGANDHA

SWEET BASIL

JAMAICA DOGWOOD

SKULLCAP

LEMON GRASS

MISTLETOE

CALIFORNIA POPPY

LAVENDER

GREAT MULLEIN

HEATHER

CATNIP

VERVAIN

CHAMOMILE

COWSLIP

CONTACT PATTI ROBERTS.

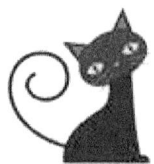

JOIN UP FOR PATTI'S NEWSLETTER:
http://bit.ly/PattiRobertsNewsletter
Twitter: http://bit.ly/1szIGfI
Facebook: http://on.fb.me/1waO1jO
Goodreads: http://bit.ly/1tdwu8f

For a complimentary copy of eBooks 1 and 2 in the Witchwood Estate Series email pattiroberts7@gmail.com with Witchwood Estate Series in the subject line.

I hope you have enjoyed reading this edition of Witchwood Estate Collectables. If you have, please leave a short review to help others find the book.

Make sure you join my newsletter and be kept up to date on new releases, special promotions, and freebies.
http://bit.ly/PattiRobertsNewsletter

ABOUT THE AUTHOR.

PATTI ROBERTS was born in Brisbane Australia but soon moved to Darwin in the Northern Territory. Her son Luke was born in 1980. Her son and grandsons are the three leading men in Patti's life. She currently lives in Cairns, Queensland, where she is writing the Paradox Series of books. Since then, Patti has commenced writing the Witchwood Estate series, and a contemporary romance, About Three Authors – Whoever Said Love Was Easy? Patti has also published a non-fiction book, Surviving Tracy, featuring real stories from survivors of Cyclone Tracy which devastated Darwin in the Northern Territory in 1974.

Patti's books are available worldwide from, libraries, bookstores on request, and all the better online stores.

You can contact Patti direct at pattiroberts7@gmail.com

Books to look out for:
Little Book Of Smoothies: For when your mojo needs a boost! (Witchwood Estate Collectables 4) http://amzn.to/2DkR6K1

KLA2EEN – A sci-fi series. We are not alone in the universe.
I'm That Girl. Contemporary drama/romance.
Girl Returned – Romance sci-fi novel about alien abduction.
Stupid Crazy – Contemporary drama/romance.
Paradox – Breathe, book 6
Witchwood Estate – Heart Bound, book 6

In her spare time, Patti designs book covers and formats for authors.
https://www.facebook.com/ParadoxBookCoversAndFormatting/